W9-CDA-828

# THE
# **SCLERODERMA**
# BOOK

# THE
# SCLERODERMA
# BOOK

*A Guide for Patients and Families*

Revised Edition

**Maureen D. Mayes, M.D.**

OXFORD
UNIVERSITY PRESS

2005

# OXFORD
### UNIVERSITY PRESS

Oxford University Press, Inc., publishes works that further
Oxford University's objective of excellence
in research, scholarship, and education.

Oxford   New York
Auckland   Cape Town   Dar es Salaam   Hong Kong   Karachi
Kuala Lumpur   Madrid   Melbourne   Mexico City   Nairobi
New Delhi   Shanghai   Taipei   Toronto

With offices in
Argentina   Austria   Brazil   Chile   Czech Republic   France   Greece
Guatemala   Hungary   Italy   Japan   Poland   Portugal   Singapore
South Korea   Switzerland   Thailand   Turkey   Ukraine   Vietnam

Published by Oxford University Press, Inc.
198 Madison Avenue, New York, New York 10016
www.oup.com

Library of Congress Cataloging-in-Publication Data
Mayes, Maureen D.
The scleroderma book : a guide for patients and families /
Maureen D. Mayes.— Rev. ed.
p. cm.
Includes bibliographical referneces and index.
ISBN-13: 978-0-19-516940-9
ISBN-10: 0-19-516940-9
1.  Scleroderma (Disease)—Popular works.  I. Title.
RL451.M39 2005
616.5'44—dc22
2004010878

1  3  5  7  9  8  6  4  2
Printed in the United States of America
on acid-free paper

This book is dedicated to
my family for their loving support.

This book is also dedicated to my patients
in gratitude for all they have taught me over the years.

# CONTENTS

✳ ✳ ✳

# PREFACE
✳ ✳ ✳

This book is meant for patients and their families who would like to know more about the disease of scleroderma. I do not expect people to read it from cover to cover, but suggest that individuals read the chapters that seem most relevant to them and to keep it as a reference when more questions or new issues arise.

Many patients find it difficult to talk about their disease to their friends and family members, since they themselves lack a medical background and are afraid of getting the facts "wrong." Others cannot bring themselves to talk to loved ones about the possible complications that could develop. On the other side of this communication gap are family members who feel left out of the picture, not even knowing what questions to ask. I hope that by sharing the information in this book, people find it easier to talk about these issues.

I also hope that this book can help to explain some of the medical terminology and make the entire process more understandable and less intimidating. Modern medicine is a complex system of specialists and procedures with a peculiar vocabulary all its own.

As I sat down to write these chapters, I simply imagined a patient sitting in front of me asking me what I was talking about. In the years I have been treating scleroderma patients, starting in 1981, I think I have gotten better about explaining what the disease is and what it does. I hope you agree.

# THE
# **SCLERODERMA**
# BOOK

# I

# INTRODUCTION TO TERMS AND TYPES OF SCLERODERMA

# 1

✳ ✳ ✳

# WHAT IS
# SCLERODERMA?

This book will tell you a lot about scleroderma. But there are two things it cannot tell you: the cause of scleroderma and the cure. These are the two most important things about any disease, and it is upsetting to the patient and frustrating for the physician that there are no clear answers to the most basic questions: "How did I get this?" and "How do I get rid of this?"

However, to say there is no cure for scleroderma is not to say that there are no effective treatments. There are many medications that can relieve the symptoms of scleroderma and others that can slow down the progression of the disease. In addition, there are new therapies under investigation that hold the promise of actually halting the disease. Although a "cure" remains elusive, the pace of medical research both directly in scleroderma as well as in related fields has accelerated tremendously in recent years. Progress in research occurs in slow and tedious steps. What appears to be a sudden breakthrough may actually be a small step that puts everything else in clear prospective. Breakthroughs are unpredictable in the short term, but inevitable in the long term.

In this introductory chapter, I will present an overview of scleroderma and introduce some technical terms. I encourage you to get familiar with these terms because they will appear throughout the book and because you will encounter them over and over again in your doctor's office and in literature about this disease. Learning the language is the first step to understanding.

### What is Scleroderma?

Scleroderma is an autoimmune connective tissue disease affecting small blood vessels and causing excess collagen accumulation. One form (localized) tends to affect children, while the other (systemic) usually affects adults, although there are exceptions to this general rule. As you will learn, scleroderma is a disease characterized by exceptions.

Scleroderma can vary a great deal in terms of severity. For some individuals it is merely a nuisance; for others it is a life-threatening illness. My youngest patient was two years old when she developed the first "spot" that turned out to be morphea (a form of localized scleroderma). My oldest patient died at 96. She had been diagnosed with the systemic form of the disease more than 50 years before. Between these two extremes of age are thousands of different stories and many different outcomes. No two stories are alike because the disease is expressed differently in different people and people respond in different ways. As with most things in life, there is no one "right" way to deal with this type of chronic illness. The purpose of this book is to give you information to demystify the disease, to give you a vocabulary to use when you discuss it with your family and with your doctor, and to help put you back in charge. This material is not meant to frighten you. If you are the type of person who sees herself or himself in all the worst scenarios, perhaps this book is not for you. If you are the type of person who is looking for answers, who feels that the way to get control is to learn as much as you can about your situation and to play an active part in your treatment, then please read on.

### *Classifying Scleroderma*

In general, diseases are classified as (1) infectious, caused by organisms like bacteria or viruses, (2) genetic or inherited, caused by a defective gene and passed down from one generation to the next, (3) malignant or cancerous, (4) degenerative, referring to changes that come with aging, and (5) autoimmune, which means that the immune system is activated to attack the body's own tissue, rather than attacking an outside organism.

Scleroderma is classified as an autoimmune disease. This puts it in the same category as lupus (systemic lupus erythematosus, or SLE), rheumatoid arthritis, Sjogren's syndrome, multiple sclerosis (MS), and several others. The causes of all these diseases are unknown and none is curable, but all are treatable.

**Table 1**    **Types of Scleroderma**

*Scleroderma*

A. Localized scleroderma (not involving internal body systems)
   1. Morphea
   2. Linear scleroderma
   3. Scleroderma en coup de sabre

B. Systemic scleroderma (involving internal systems)
   1. Limited scleroderma (sometimes called CREST)
   2. Diffuse scleroderma
   3. Scleroderma sine sclerosis

*Sclerodermalike Conditions*

A. Eosinophilic fascities (EF)

B. Scleroderma or scleromyxedema

C. Chronic graft versus host disease (GVHD)

D. Eosinophilic myalgic syndrome (EMS)

The term scleroderma means "thick skin." There are two kinds of scleroderma: the systemic form, which affects the internal organs or internal systems of the body as well as the skin, and the localized form, which affects a specific area of skin (see Table 1). There are also some conditions that are classified as sclerodermalike disorders because they share some features that are similar to scleroderma but have other features that are distinctly different.

As noted earlier, children with scleroderma usually get the localized form (further subdivided into linear scleroderma and morphea), while adults usually get the systemic form. There are exceptions to this rule, which will be dealt with in a later section.

In systemic scleroderma, the activation of the immune system causes damage to two main body parts: the small blood vessels (called the vascular system) and the collagen-producing cells located throughout the body but concentrated in the skin. In systemic scleroderma the small blood vessels tend to narrow, and sometimes the blood channel is totally closed. This is most marked in the fingers, which become overly sensitive to the cold as a result of the diminished blood supply. Small cuts on the hands are extremely slow to heal, and sometimes ulcers occur spontaneously.

Patients with systemic scleroderma are notoriously cold-sensitive (leading to thermostat wars in some households). It is this vascular part of the disease that is responsible for Raynaud's phenomenon (color changes of the fingers related to cold exposure), which happens in almost everyone (95 percent) with the systemic form of the disease. It is also this vascular abnormality that is responsible for sudden rises in blood pressure that can lead to kidney damage (about 25 percent of patients). However, it is the collagen part of the disease that is responsible for the thick and tight skin, the lung and heart problems, and the gastrointestinal features of the disease.

In contrast, localized scleroderma affects the collagen-producing cells of some areas of the skin and usually spares the internal organs and blood vessels. Localized scleroderma can occur as a single patch of thick skin, as multiple patches, as a long line of thickened skin along an arm, leg, or the forehead, or as some combination of these.

### *Collagen*

What is collagen? Collagen is a natural protein that is made by cells and deposited outside of the cell. It is what makes your skin firm, and it is the major component of connective tissue. Connective tissue is skin, tendons, joints, ligaments, and "capsules" around organs—it is what holds you together. When you get a cut, collagen is laid down to form the scar. If you have ever had a severe case of pneumonia that damaged lung tissue, the involved area of lung will heal with scar formation that can usually be seen on a chest X-ray forever. This scar formation is an essential repair process of the body.

The problem in scleroderma is that cells start making collagen as if there were some injury that needs to be repaired, even though no such injury has occurred. And once started, the cells don't turn off. In systemic scleroderma this happens first in the skin, and then can occur in the lungs, the gastrointestinal tract, the muscles, and elsewhere in the body. This excess collagen gets in the way of normal functioning. The fingers don't bend well because of the collagen buildup in the skin; the lungs can't exchange oxygen for carbon dioxide effectively because there is a thick layer of collagen where a very thin membrane is supposed to be; the esophagus and bowels can't move effectively because there is scar tissue where muscle fibers are supposed to be. Scar tissue in the heart can interfere with the usual electrical conduction system and cause an irregular or slow heartbeat. Sometimes this can be corrected with an artificial pacemaker.

Turning off these cells without damaging normal collagen formation is tricky. Under normal circumstances a small amount of new collagen is constantly being made while some old collagen is broken down. Laboratory researchers have successfully blocked all collagen production in laboratory animals, but the animals died. This is clearly not the answer. Slowing down collagen synthesis, enhancing collagen breakdown, or preventing the cells from becoming activated in the first place are approaches that are more promising. There is a great deal of research that is being done in these areas, but a safe and effective treatment strategy is yet to be found. If we knew the cause of scleroderma—that is, if we knew the trigger that started the whole process—then new treatments could be targeted to that early event. The situation is further complicated by the fact that there may be multiple triggering events that are different for different individuals. Since these causes are unknown, doctors attempt to interrupt the disease process at various levels. These treatments can slow down the progression of the disease and can even arrest it in some patients.

Localized scleroderma is a much different condition. Excess collagen production is still the underlying problem, but it occurs as one or more patches of thick, tight skin anywhere on the body. This form is called morphea. In most cases, the patch or patches develop over a period of three to five years. After that, they tend to fade and the skin texture returns to normal, although there may be some pigment differences marking the old morphea areas as lighter or darker than the surrounding normal skin. In addition, the normal layer of fatty tissue just under the skin tends to thin in the areas of morphea, so the affected leg or arm can look "thinner" than the opposite side. Usually, this difference is subtle from a distance.

The other form of localized disease is called linear scleroderma. This is an area of thickened and tight skin that develops in a "line" down one arm or leg or occasionally on the face. Usually only one limb is affected. The tissue underneath this linear scar tends to waste away, and the scar can become very deep, extending down to the muscle or bone. When it appears on an arm or leg in a young child, it can interfere with growth of the limb. Sometimes there is an inflammation of the joints (swelling and soreness) under the scar as well. Frequently, people with linear scleroderma will have a few scattered spots of morphea as well. Although this type of scleroderma usually affects children, adults can develop it too in the absence of systemic problems. Actually, it is quite rare for those with localized scleroderma to have any internal organ involvement or even to have Raynaud's phenomenon. Because of this, treatment approaches are different for localized and diffuse disease.

# 2

**❋ ❋ ❋**

# LOCALIZED
# SCLERODERMA

## *Limited, Localized, Diffuse, Generalized, Systemic, and Not-So-Systemic: What's In a Name?*

**S**cleroderma is divided into several different types, and the terminology can be confusing even to medical professionals.

### *Types of Scleroderma*

A. Localized scleroderma (not involving internal body systems)
   1. Morphea
   2. Linear
   3. Scleroderma *en coup de sabre*
B. Systemic scleroderma (involving internal systems)
   1. Limited
   2. Diffuse
   3. Scleroderma sine sclerosis

It is easy to confuse localized and limited scleroderma—and sometimes even doctors get confused by these terms, since they certainly sound similar. But they refer to very different forms of the disease. I would much prefer that the entire terminology be changed for greater clarification, but I don't make the rules. This chapter will deal with localized scleroderma, and chapters 3 and 4 will discuss the systemic form.

### What Is Localized Scleroderma?

The word *localized* is used to indicate that this form of scleroderma is confined to a specific area of skin and does not affect internal organ systems. Localized scleroderma is more common in children than in adults but can occur in both. In my practice (which is mostly adults) the youngest child I have seen with morphea (a type of localized scleroderma) was three years old, although it can start in the first few months of life. My oldest morphea patient was 86 when it started and is now over 90. I mention this older patient to make two points: first, to give a sense that scleroderma can occur in all age groups, and second, as a reminder that when doctors employ terms such as "usually" or "for the most part," you have to keep in mind that there can be exceptions. Many of my patients get alarmed when they read medical information that seems to contradict their own experiences. They conclude that what has happened to them is not supposed to happen. To help put this into a nonmedical and perhaps more universal context, everyone understands the concept that it usually does not snow in

Houston, Texas. However, sometimes it does. And with scleroderma, it can seem as if there are more cases with exceptions than those that follow the rules.

Morphea is a condition in which there are patches of thickened skin. These patches can range in size from half an inch to several inches and can occur anywhere on the body. Sometimes there is a burning, itching, or stinging sensation that happens when they first develop but frequently they are painless. The skin coloration is different from the surrounding normal skin, either lighter than normal (hypopigmented) or darker than normal (hyperpigmented). The initial spot is frequently dismissed by patients as a bruise from some minor injury that never went away. Only after it becomes noticeably thickened, or when another spot develops, is it brought to the attention of a physician. Sometimes there is only one spot, but frequently there are several, which develop gradually over a period of months or years. In some cases of morphea, and in most cases of linear scleroderma, there is a loss or "atrophy" of the layer of fatty tissue underlying the affected skin. This can cause a "sunken" appearance to the lesions.

The "typical" course of morphea in a child is that the spots develop over two to three years, then stabilize, then slowly resolve over the next few years. At their worst, the areas are thick and noticeably different from surrounding skin. As they become inactive, the skin patches return to normal texture, and by adulthood there is only a subtle difference in skin color that marks the place where the old morphea spots used to be.

This scenario is different in morphea that occurs in adults and in generalized morphea.

## Scenario 1:
### Adult Patients with inactive Childhood Morphea

Since I am trained in adult medicine, rather than pediatrics, I rarely see children. On occasion I see patients now in their twenties who come because they want a second opinion about their childhood morphea. The history usually is that their parents first noticed a spot when they were three or four years old, and it was subsequently diagnosed as morphea. By the time I see them, the spots are faded but still "findable." The issues at their visit are the following: (1) will the morphea reactivate (the answer is usually no), and (2) are they at risk to develop systemic scleroderma or another autoimmune disease like lupus (the answer is again no).

## Scenario 2:
### Active Morphea in Childhood

The milder cases of childhood morphea do not need to be treated, because the treatments have potentially serious side effects. If the morphea is spreading, with multiple spots, or if linear scleroderma is associated with it, then treatment is an option. Although clinical studies have not proven any medication to be uniformly effective in this condition, some patients seem to improve with the use of one or more types of treatment. Treatment can include the use of creams or ointments such as steroids (cortisone or cortisonelike medications), or the injection of steroids into the morphea spots. Methotrexate has been reported to be helpful. This medication is given in pill form once a week for several months or years until the scleroderma skin changes stop progressing. Methotrexate has been approved to treat rheumatoid arthritis both in adults and in children. However, blood tests have to be done periodically (monthly at first, and then less frequently) to monitor for potential side effects such as low blood counts or liver toxicity. These changes are reversible if caught early, but the need for blood-test monitoring emphasizes the fact that this medication has potential dangers. As with all medication, particularly in children, the risks must be weighed against the potential benefits. Not everyone responds to this type of treatment.

## Scenario 3:
### Morphea that Begins in Adulthood

I have seen the onset of morphea in individuals from the late teens to age 86. Most of the people I have seen have been bothered with a burning, itching, stinging sensation that signals a new lesion or the spread of an already existing one. Sometimes this feeling will begin before the skin appears abnormal, so they will know when a new spot or lesion is about to develop or when a preexisting lesion will enlarge. (The medical term *lesion* refers to any tissue abnormality, so there are skin lesions, lung lesions, brain lesions, benign lesions, cancerous lesions, and so on. It is a very general expression.)

About 50 percent of adult morphea patients, and about 20 percent of childhood patients, will have a positive ANA (antinuclear antibody) blood test. An antibody is a protein that the immune system makes that usually attaches to bacteria or viruses and helps to eliminate them from the body. It is not known why some people make an antibody to part of their own cells (the nucleus), but this is characteristic of the autoimmune diseases, particularly scleroderma and lupus.

*Table 2*   **Distincitons Between Localized and Systemic Scleroderma**

| Localized Scleroderma | Systemic Scleroderma |
| --- | --- |
| No Raynaud's phenomenon | Raynaud's phenomenon in 95 percent |
| No fingertip ulcers | Digital ulcers in more than 50 percent |
| GI involvement rarely, except for generalized morphea | GI involvement in 85 percent |
| Positive ANA in 30 percent | Positive ANA in 80 percent |

Morphea usually has no Raynaud's phenomenon (color changes of the fingers on cold exposure), a hallmark of systemic scleroderma. Additionally, there is no fingertip ulceration and no pulmonary or kidney problems, and only rarely are there any gastrointestinal problems. When GI problems do occur, they tend to be mild. For a comparison of localized and systemic scleroderma, see Table 2. The treatment approach is the same for both adults and children, that is, steroid creams or injections or methotrexate pills.

## Scenario 4:
### Generalized Morphea

Generalized morphea is a condition in which most of the skin is involved, with patches of thickened and tight skin. These patches can be so extensive that they merge into one another. The patches usually start on the trunk or upper arms and legs and then spread down to the hands and feet. This is a pattern opposite to that seen in systemic scleroderma, which starts in the hands or feet and then spreads toward the central body.

Internal organ involvement is seen more frequently in generalized morphea than in simple morphea. It particularly affects the gastrointestinal tract, causing gastroesophageal reflux (heartburn symptoms), and less frequently causes lung and kidney problems. The ANA blood test is frequently positive. Since these complications are similar to the internal organ involvement in systemic scleroderma, I will refer readers to those sections. Diagnosis is usually made by skin biopsy and by the clinical appearance of the lesions.

## Linear Scleroderma

The thickened skin of localized scleroderma can occur in patches (morphea) or along a line (linear pattern) on the head or down an arm or leg. Unlike morphea, linear scleroderma affects not just the skin and fatty tissue under the skin surface, but also underlying muscle and bone. This is particularly troublesome in growing children.

If the line of sclerodermatous skin passes over a joint, for example, the knee or the ankle, it can limit the motion of the joint and lead to limb shortening. This is, of course, more of a problem in the leg and foot than in the arm, since leg length discrepancies and limited ankle motion can severely affect gait.

In almost all cases, linear scleroderma affects only one limb. Due to the potential of leg length discrepancies and gait problems, linear scleroderma of the lower extremity is usually treated. As noted above, there are no well-designed studies that prove the effectiveness of treatment. There are reports that suggest that methotrexate may be helpful, as well as injected steroids. Other treatment approaches include physical therapy to maintain range of motion and muscle strength, splinting of a joint to prevent contracture, and in some cases surgery to improve the contracture. Contracture is a permanent bending of a joint so that it loses part of the range of motion. In scleroderma, contractures of the fingers result in bending in of the fingers toward the palm, or bending in of the elbow so the arm cannot be fully straightened out, or bending of the knee that interferes with walking. As in morphea, linear scleroderma will go through an active phase, then stabilization, then a recovery phase in which the skin returns to a more normal texture. However, the contracture tends to remain and growth does not "catch up" in the affected limb. Also, the underlying fatty tissue tends not to return to normal, so that the involved limb may always be smaller in circumference than the uninvolved limb. Fortunately, the difference is fairly subtle in many cases.

When linear scleroderma involves the head, it may take the form of scleroderma *en coup de sabre* (cut of the saber). Usually this starts as an indentation on the forehead or at the frontal hairline. Some hair may fall out in the area where the scalp is thickened. The line of thickened skin on one side of the face may only affect the forehead or it may spread down to the chin. It does not continue down the body. There may be loss of the fatty tissue under the skin on the side of the face where the linear scleroderma is. This loss of tissue or atrophy of the face is "Parry-Romberg" syndrome or "Parry-Romberg's" hemifacial atrophy. It is named after the two doctors who first described this condition in the nineteenth century: Parry and Romberg. Unfortunately, there is very little research into treatment for this condition.

Linear scleroderma can present different problems in adults, for whom growth is not an issue. The following case history, of a patient I'll call D. Q. (not his real initials), describes a fairly typical case.

D. Q. first developed painful swelling in his left knee at the age of 34. There had been no injury, and at first the concern was that his condition might be the beginning of rheumatoid arthritis. The knee pain improved with arthritis medicine, but then he developed a reddened area of skin over his left ankle. This gradually spread up the left leg. Over the course of a year, the thickened skin over his ankle limited motion, and the skin over his knee was so tight he couldn't fully bend the knee. He could straighten out the knee normally and was able to walk fairly well, but he had trouble running due to the restricted ankle motion.

Over the next three years, thickened skin developed on his thigh, with patches also on his abdomen (a combination of linear scleroderma and patches of morphea). With treatment, which included low-dose prednisone and methotrexate, the signs of inflammation resolved and the skin gradually became thinner and more elastic. Range of motion at the ankle and the knee returned to normal, although the circumference of his left calf is an inch-and-a-half smaller than the right calf. Also, the skin of the left leg is somewhat darker than the right.

At its worst, which was about two years after the onset of the disease, D. Q. developed muscle fatigue in the left leg and an aching sensation at the end of the day. Four years later, he is in the resolution phase of the disease and is able to play 18 holes of golf. He feels that the left leg is still not as strong as the right, but he has no limitations on his activities either at work or during recreation. He has no internal organ involvement, although his ANA test is positive.

The arthritis in his knee never came back. It was present only at the onset of the linear scleroderma. Although this case is somewhat unusual in that the joint swelling started before the skin lesions, the overall course, from the onset of the first skin lesion (with signs of inflammation, including redness and discomfort), an initial phase of spreading skin involvement that lasted about two years, and then slowly resolved leaving permanent loss of subcutaneous fatty tissue (the left leg is smaller than the right), is pretty typical. Did the medication do any good? When the dose was lowered, in an attempt to take him off it, the skin worsened. It then improved when the dose was increased again. Now that the skin is better, he has been able to stop all medication without a flare-up of his disease. The localized scleroderma seems to have run its course.

Although not everyone is this lucky, this is a fairly typical scenario for linear scleroderma in adults.

# 3

## \* \* \*

# SYSTEMIC
# SCLERODERMA—
# DIFFUSE

The next two chapters will deal with the systemic forms of scleroderma, both diffuse and limited, as well as scleroderma sine sclerosis, in which there is internal organ involvement but no thickening of the skin (sine means without and sclerosis means hardening).

The term *systemic* means that this form of scleroderma affects the internal organ systems. (Many textbooks use the terms *systemic sclerosis* and *systemic scleroderma* interchangeably.) The terms *limited* and *diffuse* refer to the extent of skin involvement. Both forms are associated with internal organ damage, but the limited form tends to result in less severe organ problems than the diffuse form.

Limited scleroderma sometimes occurs as the CREST form. This is an acronym that stands for calcinosis, Raynaud's phenomenon, esophageal dysfunction, sclerodactyly, and telangiectasias—features that sometime occur together. The CREST features, however, can also be seen in some individuals with diffuse skin disease, so the term *CREST* is not very useful for dividing systemic scleroderma into two separate groups. The following sections will deal with each of these features.

### *Primary Raynaud's Phenomenon*

Raynaud's phenomenon (also known as Raynaud's disease or Raynaud's syndrome), is a condition in which the fingertips turn colors on cold exposure. Typically the fingertips first turn pale, then bluish or purplish, and then redder than usual as they warm up. (In the United States, this is sometimes referred to humorously as "patriotic" color changes.) The color changes start to happen within seconds or minutes of cold exposure, and color returns to normal when the fingers are warm again. The fingers are usually numb for a period of time at the coldest point, and the patient sometimes feels a burning sensation as they warm up. Raynaud's phenomenon by itself (without scleroderma or lupus or other connective tissue disease) is very common, affecting about 5 percent of the adult American population. It is considered a "benign" condition, that is, one that is annoying but not disabling. I have even known some people with Raynaud's phenomenon in which the problem disappeared as mysteriously as it came. Many people who have it don't bother mentioning it to others, since they see themselves as unusually cold-sensitive rather than ill.

I remember being on vacation in Maine one summer with another family. We were swimming in a lake that was pretty chilly, and I remarked, rather cautiously, to my friend that her fingers appeared a little blue. I did not want to alarm her and I don't like making casual diagnoses, but it was a classic Raynaud's attack. She said she had Raynaud's, and not to worry about it, that her fingers always turned colors in the cold, and that her doctor had run some tests and said it was nothing to be alarmed about. I left it at that, because I thought her physician was correct; she did not have any of the hallmarks of scleroderma. Primary Raynaud's phenomenon does not cause sores or ulcers on the fingertips, is not associated with tight or thick skin, and really is something not to be alarmed about. If an individual has had Raynaud's phenomenon for two to five years and nothing else has developed, then it becomes extremely unlikely that an autoimmune or connective tissue disease will ever develop.

### Secondary Raynaud's Phenomenon

Secondary Raynaud's phenomenon is a different story. A typical scenario in scleroderma is that Raynaud's phenomenon develops first and the person dismisses it, thinking it is just cold sensitivity. A year or two may go by without the person bringing it to the attention of a physician, especially if she or he feels otherwise healthy. Then, in a particularly cold period, a small fingertip sore may develop that just doesn't seem to heal. Everyone knows how tender a paper cut on a fingertip can be, and that it takes days for the cut to heal and the tenderness to go away. Well, these sores, although quite small—almost the size of a pinpoint—can take weeks to heal. This is the time when many people will go to their doctor. Frequently the skin over the fingers is already shiny and a little thick, but this process is so gradual that many people overlook it.

The diagnosis of Raynaud's phenomenon is usually made on the basis of the patient's description of the typical color changes and the fact that they occur suddenly after a short period of cold exposure. Some doctors will immerse the patient's hand in ice water in an effort to provoke an attack, but I think this is somewhat cruel and unnecessary. Frequently it is unsuccessful, too, since total body cooling is usually required for an attack to occur. Most often I see patients after they have been sitting in the waiting room for a while and have had a chance to warm up, but sometimes I'll see someone who has just come in from the cold. Then I'll bring in the medical students and the residents and tell them to look at the fingers and give me a diagnosis without talking to the patient (I only do this with patients I know). One of the great delights in being a medical-school professor is that I get to stump the students—all in the name of medical education, of course.

### Limited Scleroderma

Continuing the scenario outlined above, we see the onset of Raynaud's phenomenon occurring first, followed by the gradual development of puffy fingers and/or subtle changes in the skin of the fingers with some skin thickness (for example, rings get tight and may need to be resized). Often, this is brought to the attention of a doctor only when a small fingertip sore develops that is slow to heal. This process may unfold over two to five or more years. Characteristically, an individual will also notice heartburn on a frequent, usually daily, basis.

Heartburn is a symptom of stomach acid coming up into the esophagus, a process called gastroesophageal reflux. It is felt as a burning sensation in the lower part of the chest, at the base of the breastbone (sternum). Most people have experienced heartburn after eating spicy food or a little too much food. Any woman who has been pregnant knows what heartburn feels like, as it is common in the last three months of pregnancy, especially on bending over or lying down, which causes the pregnant uterus to push on the stomach, forcing stomach acid to back up into the esophagus. Heartburn is such a common symptom that it is frequently overlooked by the patient and sometimes dismissed by a doctor or diagnosed as peptic-ulcer disease. Many doctors will not think of scleroderma when a patient comes in complaining of frequent heartburn since heartburn is common while scleroderma is rare.

Going back to our typical patient, we'll say she first noticed the color changes of Raynaud's phenomenon in 1999. Her fingers became puffy in 2001 and she began to have heartburn more frequently, causing her to start taking Tums on a regular basis. In 2003 she goes to her doctor because she has a sore on her finger that has been present for two months and just will not heal. Overall she feels pretty well, is going to work every day, and does not have the impression that she is particularly sick. All she wants is an antibiotic or some cream to help heal the sore. What she gets, however, is a lot of questions, blood tests, and a referral to a specialist who will pursue a diagnosis of a connective-tissue disease.

## *Diffuse Scleroderma*

The situation is quite different for someone with diffuse scleroderma. The onset is faster and people usually do feel ill. Raynaud's phenomenon may not be the first symptom and, in fact, may never occur. It is hard to describe a single scenario that covers the onset of diffuse scleroderma, since there is a great deal of variation, so I will describe some general patterns of onset: (1) swollen hands and feet, (2) arthritis, (3) hypertension and renal failure, and (4) gradual development of thick skin over the limbs and trunk.

### *Swollen Hands and Feet*

In this pattern, scleroderma starts with the swelling of the hands and feet. Many conditions other than scleroderma can cause swelling, or edema, particularly kidney problems and heart problems such as congestive heart failure. Additionally, some people will get foot and ankle swelling in hot weather, and many women notice some fluid retention resulting in puffy fingers just prior to their periods. Consequently, scleroderma is not the first thing a doctor will think of when a patient comes into the office complaining of swollen hands and feet. It can be a puzzling problem when all the tests are normal and no apparent cause is found. People are usually given diuretics, or "water pills," as a temporizing measure. It is a baffling situation if there are no other symptoms at this point of scleroderma, that is, if the skin texture of the hands and feet is normal (as is frequently the case in this stage), and there is no heartburn or other symptom of gastrointestinal or pulmonary (lung) involvement.

Frequently at this stage, people will have symptoms of carpal tunnel syndrome. Carpal tunnel syndrome is caused by pressure on the median nerve as it goes through a narrow "tunnel" at the wrist on the palm side. Symptoms include a tingling kind of numbness of the first three fingers that usually occurs at night and can awaken people from sleep. This numbness can also happen during the day and is relieved by shaking the hands. It is different from the numbness of Raynaud's phenomenon in that it is not triggered by cold exposure and it is not associated with color changes of the fingertips.

Carpal tunnel syndrome can develop from a variety of causes, and is frequently due to repetitive movements from working a machine or from typing. In severe cases surgery may be necessary. For those with carpal tunnel syndrome due to early scleroderma, the surgery may help the nighttime numbness, but it has no effect on the swelling. In fact, the swelling is caused by a "leakiness" of the small blood vessels in the hands, a result of damage to these vessels. The cause of the damage or the triggering event is unknown.

As time goes on, either Raynaud's phenomenon develops or the skin starts to get thick and tight, which suggests the diagnosis of scleroderma.

## Arthritis

Some cases of scleroderma start out as swollen, painful joints of the hands, wrists, and other parts of the body. As you can imagine, this lands a person in a rheumatologist's office fairly quickly, and a diagnosis of rheumatoid arthritis is frequently considered, particularly if there is no thick skin and no Raynaud's phenomenon. The picture can be somewhat puzzling, since the blood test for rheumatoid arthritis (the rheumatoid factor) is usually negative, but the ANA (antinuclear antibody) test is positive. The ANA test usually, but not always, signals lupus or scleroderma. However, in rheumatology, the diagnosis and treatment is based more on the patient's symptoms than on what the blood test shows, and so a person with such symptoms is usually treated with arthritis medication and may be initially labeled "lupus" and followed closely to determine if lupus or scleroderma will evolve. Lupus is about twice as common as scleroderma, and frequently also evolves over time so a tentative diagnosis of lupus is not unreasonable at this stage.

It may be a few months or up to two years before the characteristic skin features of scleroderma develop that permit an accurate diagnosis to be made.

### Hypertension and Renal Failure

Sometimes scleroderma begins with the sudden onset of severe high blood pressure in a person with previously normal pressure and no prior diagnosis of scleroderma. The hypertension probably develops insidiously over a period of several days, and the first symptom is either a severe headache, signs of heart failure, kidney failure, or a stroke. The person is usually taken to the emergency room, where the high blood pressure is one surprise and the presence of kidney failure an even worse surprise. The key to treatment is to lower the blood pressure, which improves the kidney function. Sometimes the skin features of scleroderma develop after such an episode. In other cases, it is possible to determine that Raynaud's phenomenon had been present for a time or that some subtle changes in the skin of the fingers were present, but these signs were not considered to be important or significant.

## *Development of Thick Skin over the Limbs and Trunk*

In some cases the thickening of the skin on the hands develops in a relatively short period, followed by extension of the skin thickness over the arms, with decreased motion of the fingers and wrists, in a matter of weeks or a handful of months. The changes are clear-cut and are brought to the attention of a physician fairly promptly. Reflux (heartburn) symptoms also occur, and there may be considerable joint pain and stiffness. The individual feels ill, with decreased energy, fatigue, and generalized muscle and joint aches and pain. This is the one form of presentation in which the diagnosis of scleroderma is made quickly. It is important to begin treatment promptly, to evaluate the degree and severity of internal organ involvement, and to monitor the patient's blood pressure and lung and heart function.

Treatment will depend on the degree and severity of inflammation in various organs and will be discussed later.

## *Scleroderma Sine Sclerosis*

Scleroderma sine sclerosis is a condition in which very typical scleroderma internal organ involvement occurs in the absence of skin thickness. Raynaud's phenomenon is usually present, which helps with the diagnosis, and the

ANA is also positive. There is often a long delay (several years) between the onset of symptoms and the diagnosis of scleroderma because the main feature of the disease (thick, tight skin) is absent.

The treatment of this form of scleroderma depends on which organ system is involved, that is, the lungs, the gastrointestinal tract, the kidneys, and so on. People with this form of scleroderma should concentrate on reading the chapters that deal with their particular type of organ involvement.

### *Delay of Diagnosis*

Scleroderma patients frequently experience a delay of diagnosis of months or even years. There are many reasons for this—the fact that it is an uncommon disease that many primary-care physicians are not familiar with, the fact that it can present with mild symptoms and at first be labeled as primary Raynaud's disease or common reflux, early lupus, stress-related fatigue, or a dozen other possible diagnoses. Whatever the reason for the delay, patients are frustrated and dismayed that the medical profession can't do a better job of recognizing this serious illness. I have no comforting response for patients and no excuses for my colleagues. My strategy (and that of the scleroderma research community) to change this situation is to educate the new doctors in training, to publish articles in the medical literature, to speak at medical meetings, and to provide this book to patients.

# 4

# * * *

# SYSTEMIC
# SCLERODERMA—
# LIMITED

W e left our patient with limited scleroderma in chapter 3 at the point of being diagnosed. Let us pick up
the story there and continue with the scenario. As you re-
call, she developed Raynaud's phenomenon (color changes
of the fingers on cold exposure) in 1999, puffy fingers and
chronic heartburn in 2001, and a fingertip sore in 2003.
The sore prompted the visit to her doctor, who ordered lots
of tests (what doctors do best) and referred her to a specialist. To make the story shorter, she is sent to a rheumatologist, without first seeing a hand specialist or a vascular
specialist. By now the blood test results are known: the blood
counts are normal, the kidney function tests are normal,
the urine analysis is normal, the liver works just fine, the
thyroid is normal, the cholesterol may be up a little, but in
general the patient is fine on paper. The only test that is

not normal is the ANA (antinuclear antibody) test, the screening test for autoimmune diseases such as lupus and scleroderma. The point of going to the rheumatologist is to find out which disease it is and, therefore, what to do about it.

The rheumatologist makes the following assessment: middle-aged woman with Raynaud's phenomenon, sclerodactyly, fingertip ulcer, GERD (gastroesophageal reflux disease), and positive ANA. This certainly looks like scleroderma by the American College of Rheumatology criteria (see Appendix 1 for these criteria).

At this point there are three things that need to be done: (1) the extent of internal organ involvement needs to be determined (in lay language, more tests), (2) the diagnosis needs to be made more definitively to consider the possibility that this may be an overlap of scleroderma and other connective tissue diseases (in lay language, even more tests), and (3) the patient and family need to be told something. This last point is most important to the patient and most problematic to the physician. The patient wants definitive answers, whereas the doctor does not yet have all the information. Too much information will overwhelm the patient and may cause unnecessary anxiety. Too little information is unsatisfying and will create the impression that the doctor is uncaring or uninformed.

My approach is to confirm that it is indeed scleroderma. I find that not having a diagnosis (and therefore fearing the worst) is more anxiety producing than knowing the diagnosis. Then I tell the story of my patient with limited scleroderma who was diagnosed at age 50 and lived to the age of 95. She had already outlived two of her doctors when I first met her.. I also inform people that this is rarely genetic, that is, it rarely runs in families and it is unlikely that they will give it to their children. The rest—the specifics of treatment, the things to watch out for in the future—I put off until the results of the workup are known.

The workup usually involves the following: more precise blood tests to identify lupus and overlap conditions; pulmonary function tests; an electrocardiogram, or EKG (also known as an ECG) to evaluate heart rhythm; an echocardiogram for heart function; and a chest X-ray if none has been taken in the past year. If there is difficulty in swallowing, as determined by the sensation that food sticks halfway down, or if there has been weight loss, then a barium swallow X-ray may be done. If the patient describes heart palpitations, then a 24-hour heart monitor may be used.

A few weeks later the patient comes back to my office for the results of the tests. In many cases at this stage, the blood tests show that there is no evidence of lupus or overlap syndromes. The pulmonary function tests are either normal or show the results of smoking, not the pattern of lung involvement in scleroderma. The EKG and echocardiogram do not show any abnormalities, and the discussion with the patient revolves around management of scleroderma symptoms.

There is no cure for scleroderma. Once you get it, you always have it. The disease can go into a phase of inactivity, in which nothing seems to be worsening, although problems with Raynaud's attacks and heartburn may persist. Some patients refer to this as a period of "remission." The point of treatment in the early phase, or at any stage of the disease, is to prevent complications from occurring, to slow the progression of the disease, and to relieve symptoms. All patients are different in that they have a different pattern of symptoms, so treatment regimens will vary from one patient to the next. For the patient described above, I will suggest a typical treatment program for this stage of her disease. Later chapters go into greater detail about different organ-system involvement and the approach to treatment for each of these conditions.

Our patient described here would benefit from the following: (1) treatment for the finger ulcer and advice about dealing with the cold to minimize the Raynaud's attacks, (2) treatment for the GERD (heartburn) to make her more comfortable and to prevent ulcers and scar tissue buildup in the esophagus that can lead to trouble swallowing, and (3) information on what to look out for in the future.

Finger ulcers occur because the blood supply to the hands is decreased. This is also the cause of the Raynaud's attacks. Treatment is directed to opening up or dilating the blood vessels with a category of medication called calcium channel blockers. There are several of these on the market. Some of them are associated with side effects such as ankle swelling and light-headedness. As with most medication, the good effects have to be balanced by the potential side effects. Pentoxiphylline can be helpful in addition to the calcium channel blockers, but it needs to be taken three times a day. Low-dose aspirin (81 mg) is frequently used as well. ACE inhibitors and ACE receptor blockers (ARB's) can also be useful. These are blood-pressure medicines that can improve circulation even in the absence of high blood pressure. There are some new medications being tested in experimental trials that may help, but as of this date they are not currently on the market.

Being careful to wear gloves and to dress warmly in cold weather is commonsense advice. Some of my patients keep little packets of chemical hand warmers (available at sporting-goods stores) in their cars to keep their hands warm before the car heater warms up. There are some cars now that are equipped with heated steering wheels, an expensive but helpful gimmick. (Don't try to get the IRS to approve this as a deduction for necessary medical equipment; they do not have a sense of humor in this regard.)

It is *essential* that patients stop smoking. Nicotine and other substances in tobacco damage the small blood vessels and will only make the Raynaud's and the finger sores worse, not to mention doing damage to the lungs.

It is helpful to protect the sores by covering them with a loose Band-Aid-type cover. If an infection occurs, take an antibiotic for a week or so; it is not wise to be on antibiotics on a continuous basis, since this can result in bacteria that become resistant to medication. A dilute form of nitroglycerin ointment can be applied at the base of the finger, not around the edges of the sore, to improve blood flow. The nitroglycerine ointment can burn if it is applied directly to the sore.

Warning signs that a skin ulcer is getting infected include the following: increased redness around the sore, increased swelling, pain and drainage, or red streaks up the arm. Under most circumstances, the sores are not infected. They start because of poor blood flow and the key to healing is to improve the circulation.

For relief of the gastroesophageal reflux, there is a class of drugs called proton pump inhibitors that are extremely helpful. These medications decrease stomach acid, improve symptoms, and decrease the likelihood of ulcers. The reason to treat and prevent the reflux is not just to eliminate the symptom of heartburn, but also to decrease the possibility of breathing in stomach acid (aspiration) especially when lying down at night. Aspiration of even a tiny amount of acid can irritate the lungs and contribute to pulmonary fibrosis, or lung scarring. So, in addition to the medication, it is wise for the patient to follow antireflux precautions. These include not eating within two hours of bedtime, not lying down immediately after a meal, raising the head of the bed by about four inches, and eliminating foods that stimulate acid, such as chocolate and caffeine. There are two other medications that are sometimes used for this condition and that can help the muscles in the esophagus and stomach to move food along. They are "pro-motility" agents and are frequently used in addition to the proton-pump inhibitors.

Pulmonary fibrosis, or buildup of scar tissue in the lungs, can occur in both limited and diffuse scleroderma. It can start several years after the onset of other symptoms even in people who have otherwise stable disease. Symptoms include a dry cough and gradual development of shortness of breath with activity. Treatment can slow down or reverse the fibrosis but is most effective if the scarring is caught early. Regular pulmonary function tests, done annually or biannually, can help to monitor this. If there is a decline in lung function from baseline or from expected values, then a high resolution CAT scan of the lungs may be done to identify inflammation, and/or an echocardiogram to evaluate heart function as a possible contributor to the shortness of breath.

Kidney involvement, caused by a rapid and severe rise in blood pressure, is uncommon in limited scleroderma, but it does occur in a small percentage of patients. To be on the safe side, individuals should have their blood pressure checked periodically. This is not as important for the patient with limited scleroderma as it is for someone with diffuse disease.

After the initial diagnosis of scleroderma is made, patients need to be followed closely by their rheumatologist to monitor potential organ involvement and response to treatment. Individuals with stable limited scleroderma—that is, in whom the disease is not getting worse—should see their rheumatologist every four to six months. If new problems arise, they should be seen more frequently, of course.

# II

## EPIDEMIOLOGY: WHO GETS SCLERODERMA AND WHY?

# 5

*  *  *

## GENETIC FEATURES OF
## SCLERODERMA

### *Did You Get It from Your Parents?*
### *Can You Give It to Your Kids?*

**P**atients frequently ask whether they can give this disease to their children. My answer to this question has
changed over the past few years. For the most part, scleroderma does not run in families. But for 1.6 percent of cases,
there is another first-degree family member (parent, brother
or sister, or child) with the disease. The flip-side of this, of
course, is that 98.4 percent of individuals do not have a family history for the disease. With the human genome project
and recent advances in the field of genetics, this has become
an area of intense research. So far, this research has resulted
in more questions than answers. It is likely that there is a
genetic susceptibility to scleroderma that involves several
different genes. However, just having the "right" (or "wrong")
set of genes is not enough. There has to be something else
that happens, in order for disease to occur. In addition, there

probably is a set of additional genes that influence the severity of scleroderma and the pattern of organ involvement. But let's take a closer look at who gets scleroderma and why.

### Genes and Scleroderma

Diseases are classified as being genetic (inherited) or acquired. Inherited diseases are the result of an abnormal gene that gets passed down from one generation to the next. Acquired diseases are caused by exposure to some triggering factor that occurs at some point after birth. Some diseases occur through an interaction between an external trigger and an internal genetic predisposition.

Examples of diseases that are totally genetic (that is, passed down from one generation to the next) are sickle cell anemia, hemophilia (a bleeding disorder), and Huntington's disease (a nerve disorder). In these conditions, the only thing necessary to develop the disease is to inherit the gene. Usually these diseases become apparent in childhood, but sometimes (as in Huntington's disease) the first symptom does not occur until middle age. In the case of dominant genetic diseases, there is an obvious family history of other relatives being affected; sometimes involving several children in a single family. In the case of recessive genetic diseases, each parent carries a copy of the abnormal gene plus a copy of the normal gene. One copy of the normal gene is enough for normal function. Each parent contributes 50 percent of their genes to their offspring. Only the children who inherit both abnormal genes express the disease. In this situation, the parents appear normal, but one out of four of their children (on average) will have the abnormality. Although harder to identify than dominantly inherited diseases, recessive diseases are usually recognized when more than one child in a family is affected. Neither of these patterns are seen with scleroderma.

Some diseases are clearly acquired, like the flu. Several people in a family are affected at the same time. Since the time period is short between exposure and illness, it is clear that there is some "bug" or infectious agent that the family members are spreading among themselves.

It has become clear that some diseases require a combination of genetic predisposition and some sort of "outside" trigger. There is no obvious inheritance pattern but multicase families are found more commonly than would be expected for a rare disease. Scleroderma is considered an example of a complex genetic disease. It is obvious that people are not born with it but develop or acquire it later in life. This means that they "catch it" somehow, from being exposed to something in the environment, perhaps a virus, a bacterium, a chemical, or an allergen (an allergy-causing agent).

Many diseases are caused by a combination of genes and environment. High blood pressure, or hypertension, is a good example, as is the tendency to have heart attacks. Hypertension and heart disease frequently run in families. But even if people have the susceptibility genes, they do not have to get the disease if they are careful with their diet, exercise, take medications to keep blood pressure and cholesterol levels normal, and other sorts of measures. Many of the diseases in modern life fall into this category.

Is there a gene for scleroderma? The answer, from what we know now, is that there probably is a susceptibility gene or several susceptibility genes, without which people could not get scleroderma. However, just having the gene is not sufficient; there must be some additional trigger to make the disease happen. There are examples from other diseases that could make this theory plausible. Rheumatic fever, for instance, is caused by the streptococcus bacteria that also causes strep throat. Strep throat is very common; almost every child develops it at some point. It is usually treated with penicillin or another antibiotic, which cures the problem. However, in some individuals, strep throat is complicated by the heart damage, high fevers, and joint swelling of rheumatic fever. The joint inflammation lasts about a month and then goes away, but the heart valve damage lasts forever and tends to worsen with age. Now that penicillin and other antibiotics are commonly used to treat strep throat, the incidence of rheumatic fever in the United States is much lower than it was 50 years ago. But even before the age of antibiotics, not everybody who got strep throat developed rheumatic fever. This was a puzzle for years, and it is only recently that researchers figured out that only those people who have a particular gene will get this complication.

What is the evidence that there is any role for genes in the development of scleroderma if most individuals have no family history of this disease? The evidence comes from an unlikely source: a group of Native Americans of the Choctaw tribe in Oklahoma who have a much higher than expected prevalence of scleroderma (almost eight times the prevalence in the rest of the country). These individuals have an unusual combination of immune regulation genes that non-Choctaws in Oklahoma do not have. One of the problems with labeling this gene complex as the "scleroderma gene" is that there are Choctaws who live in the southeastern United States who have this same unusual combination of immune-regulation genes but do not get scleroderma. The answer to this riddle is either that there are other genes (as yet unidentified) that the Oklahoma Choctaws have and the southeastern Choctaws do not have, or that there is something in the environment in Oklahoma that has triggered scleroderma in this group. The search is on for these genes, but this may give us only half of the story. Of course, half of the story is a lot better than none, which is where we are now in our understanding of the cause of scleroderma.

An additional line of evidence for a genetic link comes from the few families in which more than one member is affected. Among the more than 500 scleroderma patients I've seen, there are two families with scleroderma in two related individuals. One is a brother and a sister—he has diffuse disease and she has limited disease. The other family has two sisters affected. In both these situations, the diagnosis was made years apart, and long after these people had left home, so they had not shared the same environment for years. Could this have occurred by chance alone? This is pretty unlikely. Could this have happened not because of having a "scleroderma gene" but by being exposed to a particular virus or bacterium, which then stayed dormant in the body for years before emerging as scleroderma? We just don't know. We do know that viruses can remain in the body for decades and manifest years later as a disease that is very different from the original one caused by the virus. This is the case with chicken pox and shingles. Almost every child in this country gets chicken pox. Once infected, even though the pox "spots" go away in a few weeks, the virus stays in the nerve cells in an inactive state. Decades later it can reactivate and cause shingles, a very painful line of blisters that develop along a nerve pathway. The blisters will go away, but the pain can last for many months, and another attack of shingles can occur years later.

One way to distinguish between the role of genetics and the role of environmental factors is to study twins. If a disease is strictly genetic, then both members of a set of identical twins should have the disease. If the disease is strictly due to exposure (exposure here can mean a viral or bacterial infection, as well as exposure to a chemical or toxin) and if the exposure happened after the twins grew up and left the shared home environment, each twin should have only the same chance of getting the disease as the general population. (Actually, the best way to study this is to get twins who were separated at birth and therefore do not share any of the home environment, but this is extremely difficult.)

A study of twins, both identical and fraternal (nonidentical), was done by Dr. Timothy Wright and his colleagues at the University of Pittsburgh. They gathered blood samples from as many twins as possible, at least one of whom had scleroderma. What this group of researchers found is that the identical twins, who have identical genes, were no more likely to both have scleroderma than the nonidentical twins, who are no more closely related than any other brothers and sisters, but that this likelihood among all twins was higher than the likelihood in the general population. To put numbers on this, the likelihood of both twins in a twin pair having scleroderma was 6 percent, which is higher than what occurs in the general population, but nowhere near the 100 percent that would be expected if the disease was purely genetic. The conclusion from this, as from the pattern of the disease among Oklahoma Choctaws, is that there is some genetic component in scleroderma, but that there is something else in the outside world that a person must come in contact with in order to get the disease. I will discuss what little we know about this "something else" in the next chapter.

One final note about the twin study: This is an excellent example of collaboration among scleroderma researchers. I contributed a twin pair to this study, as did many other researchers around the country. We realize that solving the mystery of scleroderma will require this kind of cooperation and are hopeful that it will produce results soon.

# 6

**✳ ✳ ✳**

# EPIDEMIOLOGY OF
# SCLERODERMA

*Numbers of Patients, Occupational
Links, and Environmental Concerns*

How many scleroderma patients are there in the United States? There has been some confusion and controversy over this number in the past. Studies of scleroderma have been hindered by the following three factors: (1) scleroderma is an uncommon condition, (2) the diagnosis can be difficult to make with certainty (the classification criteria were established only in 1980), and (3) until fairly recently there were few researchers interested in studying this disease.

Epidemiology is the study of the pattern of disease occurrence, that is, the prevalence of disease (the total number of cases) the incidence of the disease (how many new cases occur each year), and whether the condition is becoming more or less common. Epidemiologists study whether there are particular populations more likely to get a disease, for example, men versus women, one ethnic group more than another, or people in one country or geographic location more than another. By studying these patterns important risk factors for disease development can be identified providing clues to the cause or causes of the disease. In addition, knowledge of these risk factors could be used to help prevent the disease by avoiding these risks.

For systemic scleroderma (including both the limited and the diffuse forms of the disease), the prevalence is approximately 250 cases per million American adults. This comes to about 80,000 patients in the United States for the prevalence estimate of systemic sclerosis. For localized scleroderma (including morphea and all its subtypes as well as linear scleroderma), the number is probably twice that for systemic disease, but accurate figures are not available. Overall, the number of new cases of systemic scleroderma is about 5,000 each year for the annual incidence, and the number of new cases of localized scleroderma is about 6,000 each year. The number in the United States appears to be higher than that in Europe and Japan, although it is somewhat unclear if this difference is true or if it reflects differences in the methods of counting cases.

No definite answer can be given to the question of whether scleroderma is now more common than in the past, since really comprehensive studies have only been done in the past 20 years. However, in this relatively brief period, it does not seem that there are more new cases. The disease is becoming more widely known through the public relations work of scleroderma organizations and through the efforts of individual patients. This increased awareness may give the false impression that overall incidence is growing.

Women get scleroderma more frequently than men, and in fact over 80 percent of people with systemic sclerosis are women. This is also true for most forms of localized scleroderma, with the exception of linear scleroderma, which affects males and females equally. If more women get this disease, do female hormones play a role? Once again, the jury is still out. One study found that taking birth control pills did not affect the likelihood of getting scleroderma but taking female hormones to treat menopause did raise the likelihood but only slightly. These two findings seem contradictory, and it is not clear what role, if any, female hormones play in disease development. It must be noted also that there is no evidence of any hormone imbalance in male patients, so right now the fact that scleroderma is more common in women remains an observation only, without a real explanation. Both rheumatoid arthritis and lupus are more common in women than in men, but hormones appear to have different effects in these two diseases. Pregnancy usually makes the symptoms of rheumatoid arthritis better, whereas pregnancy in lupus patients frequently makes the disease worse. Pregnancy in scleroderma is considered a high-risk situation, although many patients do quite well.

There are particular ethnic groups that seem to have a higher incidence of scleroderma. The highest prevalence of systemic scleroderma is found in the Choctaw Native Americans in Oklahoma. The reason for this high disease occurrence is not completely understood, but evidence suggests that this group of people have a genetic predisposition for scleroderma. African Americans have a slightly higher risk of getting the disease than do European Americans, and this effect is most notable in younger age groups.

Also, blacks tend to have diffuse disease more frequently than whites. The reasons for this are not clear.

What about risk factors other than gender and ethnicity? Evidence for an association between scleroderma and chemicals or other materials in the environment, or particular occupations, is suggestive but not at all conclusive. Miners (coal miners in Pennsylvania and Germany, as well as gold miners in South Africa) have been reported to have an increased incidence of scleroderma. However, this does not explain the vast majority of cases, since very few women, and not too many men in the United States, are employed in mining. Out of my hundreds of patients, only one had an exposure related to mining, and this could have been coincidental.

Exposure to various chemical solvents also has been reported to be associated with scleroderma, but again, this does not account for the vast majority of cases.

It is natural for people to try to determine what caused their disease. It is very difficult psychologically and emotionally not to know the cause. It is impossible to protect your family from getting it if you can't tell them what to avoid. The past 20 years of my professional life have been involved with solving this mystery. I hope that my next 20 years will not be spent similarly and that one day scleroderma will be relegated to textbooks on the history of medicine.

# III

# HOW SCLERODERMA AFFECTS THE BODY

# 7

**❋ ❋ ❋**

# RAYNAUD'S PHENOMENON, SKIN INVOLVEMENT, AND FINGER SORES

This chapter relates to people with the systemic form of scleroderma, including both those with limited disease and those with diffuse disease. It does not apply to people with localized scleroderma, which is morphea and linear scleroderma.

### Raynaud's Phenomenon

Raynaud's phenomenon is a specific type of cold sensitivity that is characterized by color changes of the fingertips on cold exposure. There is some variation from one person to the next, but the typical Raynaud's episode starts with the fingertips getting very pale, then numb, and then turning a purple or blue color. This process starts within minutes of cold exposure and will last until the fingers get warm again. Sometimes the fingertips turn red as they warm up; this can produce a throbbing or burning sensation.

Raynaud's phenomenon is a common condition, affecting about 5 percent of the adult American population. Most of these people have primary Raynaud's phenomenon and will never develop scleroderma or other connective tissue disease. However, a small percentage of people will go on to develop scleroderma or lupus. In these people, the cold sensitivity is called secondary Raynaud's phenomenon. To make things even more complicated, some people with scleroderma do not have Raynaud's at all. However, most people with scleroderma do develop this cold sensitivity as the first sign or symptom that something unusual is happening.

The underlying process in a Raynaud's attack is a spasm of the small blood vessels in the fingers, causing the blue or purple color. The toes also are affected in many people, but the fingers are the most noticeable. These color changes are really an exaggeration of a normal response to cold exposure, since everyone will develop cold hands when they are exposed to cold for a long enough period of time. However, the normal cold response in the hands is a blotchy red and white pattern, and Raynaud's-type color changes are distinctly different.

How do you determine the difference between primary Raynaud's phenomenon and the secondary form? The distinction is made through a careful evaluation by your physician, who looks for features that would suggest either scleroderma or lupus. These include swelling of the hands, thickened skin on the fingers, difficulty swallowing, or frequent heartburn, in the case of scleroderma; or sun-sensitive skin rashes, joint problems, and other symptoms in the case of lupus. Additionally, a blood test (the ANA, or antinuclear antibody test) is usually done. The diagnosis of either scleroderma or lupus is made when the patient has a combination of physical symptoms, usually in conjuction with a positive blood test. If the workup is negative for signs and symptoms of these other diseases, and especially if the ANA is negative, then it is likely that the Raynaud's phenomenon is primary. However, sometimes it takes a while (two to five years) for the other features to develop, so most physicians will follow a patient for a few years before feeling comfortable assuring her or him that nothing else is likely to happen.

Sometimes I see people with Raynaud's phenomenon and a positive ANA, but nothing else, even after ten or more years of the typical color changes. I think these people also have primary Raynaud's phenomenon and should be reassured. The antinuclear antibody does not do anything bad by itself. It is only a marker for connective tissue disease. Also, the ANA does not distinguish between scleroderma, lupus, and mixed connective tissue disease. I wish I could explain this better, but I am hindered because not a lot is known about what makes this test positive to begin with. If it offers you any consolation, you now know almost as much about the ANA as your doctor.

### Systemic Scleroderma and the Skin

The thickened skin of scleroderma is the most noticeable feature of the disease. As noted in earlier chapters, there can be only a limited degree of skin thickening, and this small amount can be missed by many doctors who are not familiar with the more subtle changes of scleroderma. The skin thickness can be limited to the fingers (*sclerodactyly*) or can also involve the back of the hand, the forearm, the upper arm, the trunk, the legs, and the feet. It starts in the hands or feet and may or may not progress to involve other areas of the body. I have seen patients with all combinations of skin involvement. It is generally true that the skin thickening reaches its maximum extent within two to five years of the start of the thickening (not within five years of the onset of the Raynaud's changes). After a few years the thick skin can start to improve on its own even without treatment.

As noted earlier, the word scleroderma means "thick skin." The thickness comes from an excess of scar tissue, which consists of collagen. Collagen is a normal component of skin, bones, cartilage, lungs, and just about every other organ in the body. It forms a sort of scaffold in which cells and organs reside. Under ordinary circumstances, collagen is a good thing.

In order to understand the role of collagen in scleroderma, and in order to understand the abnormality in this disease, we must discuss some basic cell biology. Formation of a scar is the body's normal response to damage done by trauma. Most of us have scars from old cuts or lacerations. Even internal organs can form scar tissue as part of the repair process. An example of this is lung scarring following a severe bout of pneumonia.

The normal sequence for the repair process after a laceration or cut that penetrates through the skin (that is, through both the epidermis and the dermis) involves several steps. The first response is bleeding and clot formation to "plug" the hole. Then cells in the dermis (*fibroblasts*) become activated, actually move to the edge of the damaged tissue, and start making collagen. Under the microscope, collagen looks like a wavy rope or fiber. These fibers fill in the defect from the injury. Eventually the clot (scab) lifts off to reveal the scar underneath, and the structural integrity of the skin is restored. The activated fibroblasts either die off or return to a resting state, on guard for subsequent injuries.

How do the fibroblasts know that an injury has occurred, and how do they know where to go? This is an interesting question, because the answer to what triggers scleroderma is contained in the answer to it. While some substances, such as glucose and other nutrients, are always passing out of blood into tissue, blood is supposed to stay inside blood vessels, and fibroblasts are supposed to stay in tissue outside of blood vessels. When blood vessels are damaged, they release a large number of inflammatory substances, some of which activate fibroblasts and set in motion the repair mechanism of scar formation described above. (The white cells in the blood play a key role in releasing substances that activate fibroblasts; this is how the immune system is involved.)

In scleroderma, however, the fibroblasts become activated even though there is no apparent injury—no initial cut, no laceration. For some unknown reason and by some unknown mechanism, blood vessels spontaneously become "leaky," and skin fibroblasts start making too much collagen. This activation can occur in one or more small areas over several years (morphea). It can occur in a line down a limb (linear scleroderma), or it can occur beginning in the hands and progressing over the body, even including, to a varying extent, the internal organs (systemic scleroderma). No one knows what causes the blood vessel damage to begin with. A great deal of research has been done to identify specific factors that turn on the fibroblasts, and there is a tremendous interest in developing drugs that will block these factors and turn off the fibroblasts.

No one knows why some people get a mild case, with skin thickening only involving the fingers, while others get skin thickness and tightness over the entire body. No one knows, either, why it is that some people get severe internal organ involvement (in the lungs, GI tract, or kidneys) while others get little to none. There may well be a genetic component that determines the severity of the disease. Although I cannot answer your "why" questions, I can answer some of your "how" questions. (I have been working on the "why" question since 1981, and I am confident that the answer will eventually be found.)

Skin problems in scleroderma can be grouped into six categories: (1) itching, or pruritus, (2) pigment changes, both darker skin and patchy areas of lighter skin, (3) skin ulcers, (4) skin thickness, resulting in joint contractures, (5) hair loss, (6) telangiectasias, or red spots, and (7) calcinosis, or calcium deposits.

### Itching

Itching, also known by the medical term pruritus, is a major problem for some people. It is caused by irritation in the skin from the underlying inflammatory process associated with scleroderma. It occurs without a rash, although some individuals will get a rash from scratching. The itching is worse at night (probably because the distractions of the day are fewer) and can be bad enough to interfere with sleep. For the most part, the itching occurs in the first two to five years of the disease and then subsides, although some people have persistent problems with it for many years.

In terms of treatment, low-dose steroids (such as prednisone) can be helpful, but they have a lot of potential side effects, so this is usually considered a last resort. Antihistamines are somewhat helpful and have the added benefit of causing drowsiness. Creams and lotions may yield a temporary benefit but do not penetrate deep enough to provide prolonged relief. Some patients have reported improvement with the use of antidepressants such as Zoloft or Paxil, but there is no scientific evidence that these are effective.

### Pigment Changes

Pigment (skin color) changes occur commonly in scleroderma. Some areas may have increased pigmentation (hyperpigmentation) and appear darkened, like a tan that doesn't fade, even though there has been no sun exposure. Other areas of skin may develop a patchy loss of skin pigment (hypopigmentation) in a "salt-and-pepper" fashion. On close inspection, the areas at the base of a hair follicle can be seen to have a spot of normal pigment while the surrounding areas have lost pigment. Sometimes this is mistaken for vitiligo, a skin disorder manifested by a smooth loss of pigment. Pigment changes can present a cosmetic problem. In some cases, prescription creams containing vitamin A (usually considered acne creams) can be helpful, but it can take months for them to have an effect, and these creams can be drying. For areas of the face and neck, makeup may be the only recourse. Over several years these changes can resolve and the skin tone returns to a more normal appearance.

*Skin Ulcers*

Skin ulcers are far more than a cosmetic problem. These usually occur on the fingers, either at the tips, due to poor circulation, or over the knuckles, where the skin is stretched tight. (Toe ulcers can also occur; both kinds are usually referred to in the medical literature as digital ulcers.) Sometimes a small cut or injury to the fingertip develops into a sore that will not heal because the blood supply is not good enough. Sores can occur at pressure points—for example, over the elbows—as well. Wherever these sores occur, they are painful and interfere with function. Treatment includes medication to improve the blood supply by dilating or widening the blood vessels (vasodilators), medication to help the red cells move through narrowed blood vessels (pentoxiphylline), cold avoidance, protection from the dozens of daily small traumas that can damage the fingers, keeping the area clean and dry, and constant vigilance against infection. Infections can occur in sores that are open for a long period of time, and these need to be treated with antibiotics. Because the underlying problem is usually the lack of blood supply, rather than an infection, the antibiotics alone will not cause the sore to heal. Once an ulcer develops, it typically takes weeks or months to heal.

The best way to treat these ulcers is to prevent them from happening in the first place by being cautious about cold exposure, which further reduces the blood supply to the extremities. Always wear gloves or mittens when cold exposure is likely, even in an unlikely place such as the grocery store. At first some patients feel self-conscious, but it does not matter what other people think. In the winter many of my patients keep little packets of chemical warmers in their cars to hold in their hands until the car heater gets going. It also helps to dress warmly, with an extra sweater or undershirt. There is no medicine that will completely eliminate the Raynaud's attacks, but there are several medications that can decrease the severity and frequency of these attacks. They belong to a class of drugs called calcium channel blockers. All medications have potential side effects, so you should discuss these with your doctor.

Primary Raynaud's phenomenon can be improved with biofeedback treatment. This is a technique in which a person learns to increase the blood supply to the fingers. Although biofeedback may be less helpful in the secondary Raynaud's attacks of scleroderma, it can be beneficial for some people. It takes a lot of practice and motivation. Biofeedback is usually taught by psychologists. Briefly, a small wire that measures temperature is taped to a finger. This is connected to a gauge that indicates to the patient if the finger temperature is going up or down. The person is then instructed to try raising the temperature by imagining he or she is in a warm room, in a hot climate, and so on. The point is that with practice (usually at least ten sessions) most people can learn to raise their finger temperature. Practice is required until it becomes "automatic," so that the technique can be used on the spur of the moment. Biofeedback will not cure Raynaud's phenomenon, but in some individuals the technique can decrease the frequency and severity of attacks.

Sometimes finger ulcers occur in spite of careful precautions. In this case, it is important to be on medications to improve blood flow, to use antibiotics only if an infection has set in, and to be very careful to keep warm. Nitroglycerine cream or nitroglycerine patches can also be used.

This is the same medicine that is used to treat heart disease because it helps to open up blood vessels. The cream will burn if it is applied directly over the ulcer. It can be placed at the base of the finger but the cream tends to rub off on clothing, so I prefer the patch. A nitroglycerine patch can be placed over the back of the hand for 12 hours, usually at night, and then removed during the day, and a new patch applied the next night. Continual use of the patch can lead to "tolerance" so that the body gets used to the medicine and the effect is diminished. Also, nitroglycerine can cause headaches and lower the blood pressure, effects that diminish if people are lying down. Once the ulcer heals the patches are no longer necessary. Actually, it does not matter where on the body that the patch is placed. But I think there is a psychological advantage to placing it on the hand with the worse ulcers. I have no objection to psychological advantages as long as they are coupled with sound medical advice.

In cases of severe and recurrent ulcers, surgery can be done to help free up the tiny blood vessels at the base of the finger. This is called digital sympathectomy, and removes the sympathetic nerves that are responsible for causing the blood vessels to go into spasm. This is very delicate surgery and there may be problems with healing of the surgical incision, so this procedure is usually reserved for the more extreme cases. In very rare cases, the tip of the finger may need to be surgically amputated in order to relieve pain and remove dead or dying tissue.

In a small percentage of cases, there is a blockage in the medium-sized arteries in the forearm. For those with recurrent or multiple ulcers, an ultrasound or "Doppler" test of the blood flow in the arm should be done to look for this type of block. Another test called an angiogram may be needed to pinpoint the location and severity of the block. An angiogram is a test in which a dye is injected into the artery above the block and an X-ray of the arm and hand is done as the dye moves down the arteries into the hand. If a block is identified, surgery may be needed to bypass it. However, most patients do not have any problems with the blood vessels in the upper arm or forearm. The usual cause of decreased circulation is narrowing of the small arteries in the fingers, which are too small to bypass.

Ulcers can also occur over the knuckles or over the elbows. This tends to happen due to a combination of poor blood supply, stretched skin, and "microtrauma," that is frequent small injuries to fingers that happen every day, or repeated pressure from leaning on the elbows. The measures noted above (keeping warm, keeping the area clean, treating infections if and when they happen, using medication to improve blood circulation) are very important. Ulcers that occur on the lower legs or around the ankles are likely due to a different problem in the blood vessels, called vasculitis, which is treated with a different class of medication that reduces inflammation.

### Skin Thickness Resulting in Joint Contractures

Skin thickness occurs in almost all patients with scleroderma and is the hallmark of this disease. In some individuals the extent and degree of skin thickness is fairly mild, affecting only the fingers. In those whose skin is moderately affected, there is thickness of the skin of the fingers, back of the hands, forearms, face, and lower legs. In others, thickness can involve the skin of the trunk (chest, abdomen, and back) as well as the skin of the face, arms, and legs.

In research studies of new drugs, the degree and extent of skin involvement is measured by a skin scoring system. The body is divided into areas (fingers, dorsum of the hands, forearms, upper arms, face, chest, abdomen, thighs, legs, and feet). The degree of skin involvement is determined by assigning a number (0 = normal, 1 = mild, 2 = moderate, or 3 = severe skin thickness) to each of these areas. The numbers are then added together for a total skin score. The highest or worst score is 51. If the medicine under study is effective, then the skin score is expected to improve or get lower over time. Since some people will experience spontaneous improvement in skin score over time, a placebo group (those getting a "dummy" pill that does not contain the real medicine) is needed for comparison. Statistical analysis is done to determine if the people on the real medicine experienced a greater level of improvement than the people on the placebo pill.

Another way to objectively determine if the disease is improving or worsening is to measure the degree and extent of joint contractures. Since the fingers tend to curl inward toward the palm (finger or flexion contractures) in scleroderma, the degree of hand extension is often used to gauge disease progression. This is done by having the patient extend the fingers (open the hand) as wide as possible and, using a measuring tape, measure the distance from the tip of the thumb to the tip of the little finger. This is repeated from visit to visit and provides a fairly reliable and objective measure of hand function. Most research studies of potential medicines to help scleroderma skin changes include measures of hand extension.

Not everyone with scleroderma will get flexion contractures of the fingers. Again, this is highly variable. However for those with the contractures, a common problem is the development of ulcers over the bent knuckles due to frag-ile "stretched" skin. The same measures of keeping warm, using medicine to improve the circulation and protecting against injury are important. If these are unsuccessful, there is a surgical approach that can be helpful. The surgery in-volves removing the finger joint, straightening the finger, and fusing the bones with small metal pins. As you can imagine, such an operation is reserved for somewhat severe cases and should only be done by hand surgeons who are familiar with scleroderma hands. This usually means going to a sclero-derma center to have the surgery.

## Hair Loss

Sometimes the hair falls out in the areas of thickened skin over the arms and legs. This is due to increased collagen around the hair follicles in the dermis as well as to de-creased blood supply to the follicles. One of the changes that heralds improvement in scleroderma is the regrowth of hair. Hair loss from the scalp can happen as well, but this is more characteristic of lupus and overlap syndromes (lupus and scleroderma or mixed connective tissue disease) than of scleroderma alone.

## Telangiectasias

Telangiectasias are red spots caused by the dilatation (wid-ening) of small blood vessels in the skin. In scleroderma these spots tend to occur on the hands and face, but can occur all over the body. Usually they are simply a marker of scleroderma and by themselves cause no harm. Under-standably, however, people don't like them, because they don't like having red spots especially on their face. These can be removed by laser treatment, but they tend to recur.

The only situation in which medical treatment is necessary (rather than cosmetic) is if the telangiectasias become very large and bleed. In rare situations, these blood vessel malformations can occur in the mouth, throat, or stomach and cause significant bleeding problems. Laser therapy is the treatment of choice.

## *Calcinosis*

Small calcium deposits can occur in the fingers, over the elbows, over the knees, and in various other places. They start out underneath the skin and feel firm. An X-ray can confirm that they are calcium deposits (they show up as white dots) and nothing to worry about. They cause problems only if they are in certain areas of the hands or fingers and get in the way of hand function. Sometimes they break through the skin and drain a white material. If open and draining, they can become infected from the normal bacteria that live on the skin.

For the most part, I advise against surgical removal of these calcium deposits because the incision site will be slow to heal and because they tend to come back. At this point there is no good way to prevent them from occurring. It does not matter if your diet is high or low in calcium. The medications for Raynaud's condition mentioned above, the calcium channel blockers, have been suggested as a treatment, but most of my patients were already on these medications when the calcium deposits developed, so I don't think they are particularly helpful. Colchicine (a medicine usually used to treat gout) is sometimes helpful to treat the inflammation associated with these deposits.

# 8

**❋ ❋ ❋**

# SCLERODERMA
# AND THE KIDNEYS

Kidney involvement occurs in about 20 percent of scleroderma patients. While the good news is that 80 percent of patients will never get this complication, the bad news is that it is difficult to predict which 20 percent will be affected. Kidney problems occur most frequently in the first five years after the diagnosis and tend to happen in those individuals with diffuse skin involvement, that is, with skin thickness that extends to the upper arms or the trunk. Although this is generally true, scleroderma kidney disease can affect others as well. As I said before, throughout this book it will become clear that there are many exceptions to the rule when it comes to scleroderma patients.

Kidneys are damaged in scleroderma due to a sudden and severe increase in blood pressure, referred to as malignant phase hypertension, which is also called scleroderma renal crisis. This is very different from the usual kind of high blood pressure, or hypertension, which tends to start gradually and that results in organ damage such as strokes and heart attacks only after many years. In scleroderma, blood pressure can go from normal or even low normal levels to dangerously high levels in a matter of days, and kidney failure can occur in a matter of weeks. As with the "usual" type of hypertension, there are no symptoms in the early stages. After the first few days, the hypertension can cause persistent or recurrent headaches, nausea, and vomiting. If malignant phase hypertension continues uncontrolled, kidney function can be lost and can progress to total kidney failure. Once this happens, dialysis is necessary.

The way to prevent kidney damage is to detect and treat the scleroderma-related hypertension as soon as possible. Patients who are considered to be in the high-risk category should invest in a home blood pressure apparatus and measure their pressure on a regular basis. Twice a week is usually considered to be often enough. Some people find it easier to remember if they do this daily, and that of course is fine as well. There are two numbers that reflect blood pressure: the systolic number that is always the higher number, and the diastolic number. A typical blood pressure for a healthy 30-year-old woman is 110/70. In this example, the "110" is the systolic pressure and the "70" is the diastolic pressure. Most people think they only have to worry about the top number but actually both numbers are important.

If the pressure starts to go up, then it should be taken on a daily basis. If the blood pressure stays elevated for three days in a row, then your doctor should be contacted. How high is too high will depend to some extent on what a person's blood pressure normally runs. If your doctor advises you to take your blood pressure on a regular basis then find out from him/her what is the "cutoff" number that should prompt a phone call to the office.

If malignant phase hypertension occurs and is caught early, the blood pressure can be brought under control with medication, usually ACE inhibitors (angiotensin-converting enzyme inhibitors). Other types of blood pressure medications tend not to work as well as the ACE inhibitors and will not prevent the onset of this problem. If the pressure does start to go up, it is very important to get it down to normal levels as quickly as possible. This will require frequent blood tests to monitor kidney function, and adjustment of medication doses as required. Sometimes this can be done as an outpatient, but occasionally, at least with the first episode of hypertension, patients will need to be hospitalized.

Once kidney function is lost, dialysis becomes necessary to maintain life. Dialysis is a process in which blood is removed from the body and passed through a special machine that removes the waste products from the body, which the kidneys normally remove. The filtered blood is then put back into the patient. This process takes about four hours and is usually done three times a week. One of the difficulties with dialysis is that the dialysis machine does not do as good a job as normal kidneys, and people don't feel as well as normal. In some cases of scleroderma renal failure, some kidney function can be regained and the person can go off dialysis if the blood pressure is kept under control.

However, if kidney failure persists and long-term dialysis is needed, a kidney transplant can be done. There is the concern that hypertension will come back and ruin the transplanted kidney. However, the immunosuppressive medication used to prevent rejection of the kidney transplant will help to keep the scleroderma under control. And, of course, the blood pressure must be carefully monitored and controlled.

Clearly not every headache and not every episode of nausea or vomiting represents an episode of uncontrolled high blood pressure. This is why it is important to have a blood pressure cuff at home and know how to take your own pressure. For individuals who have limited scleroderma (skin tightness limited to areas below the elbows and below the knees), it is not usually necessary to take frequent blood pressures.

Once a person has had problems with scleroderma-related hypertension and gotten it under control with medication, it may be possible to decrease the dosage and in some cases go off the medication entirely. In this case, the pressure should be monitored frequently (again, twice a week). These individuals are at risk for repeated episodes of hypertension. If caught early and treated immediately, the pressure usually returns to normal and there is no damage to the kidneys. Sometimes high-risk patients are treated with ACE inhibitors even without an episode of malignant hypertension. This approach however may not prevent an episode because the dose of the ACE inhibitor has to be low in people with normal blood pressure in order to avoid lowering the pressure too much. Low doses of ACE inhibitors are probably not strong enough to prevent renal crisis. These individuals should still monitor their pressures on a regular basis.

The difficulty, as you probably have already figured out, is in promptly identifying and treating the first episode of malignant hypertension. As noted above, since this problem occurs in only a small number of patients who are at risk for several years, what is the best advice to give someone in order to strike a balance between reasonable safety and unnecessary worry? I recommend that you speak to your own doctor to find out if you are at high risk of developing this form of high blood pressure. If the answer is yes, then you should learn how to take your own pressure and find out at what pressure level you should be concerned and notify your doctor. For the most part, it will be reassuring to know that your pressure is normal.

Blood pressure usually fluctuates quite a bit on a daily basis and from day to day. For most people, the pressure is lowest in the morning and rises with activity during the day. I recommend that my high risk patients take their blood pressure around the same time every day. It really does not matter what that time is, and I give them a range of normal pressures, approximately 100–150 (systolic) over 60–90 (diastolic). A single reading of 160/92 should not cause alarm, but indicates that the pressure should be taken on a daily basis for the next few days. If the pressure stays at this level for three days in a row, especially in someone whose blood pressure is normally in the 100/60 range, then treatment should be started and the patient watched very carefully. On the other hand, if someone's blood pressure is usually 150/88, then the allowable levels will be different.

What about those people who have scleroderma and, coincidentally, have the usual kind of high blood pressure? Scleroderma is rare, but high blood pressure is very common in the United States, and the two conditions will overlap in some people just by chance. Actually, it is easy to tell the difference. Scleroderma-related hypertension occurs abruptly, and once elevated, the blood pressure continues to climb and can go to very dangerous levels that can result in a heart attack or a stroke. Also, blood tests that measure kidney function are abnormal, blood counts may be low, and a urinalysis will show protein and blood cells in the urine. Usual hypertension, on the other hand, tends to remain at about the same level day after day, and kidney function tests are normal for years.

On rare occasions, scleroderma will start with an episode of malignant phase hypertension, and the other features of scleroderma (Raynaud's phenomenon, skin thickness, GI problems) happen afterward. In such cases, there is no reasonable way to detect the problem early.

The good news in all of this is that since 1980 when ACE inhibitors first became available, scleroderma renal crisis became a treatable and reversible disease if caught early and treated promptly. Even if renal failure happens and dialysis becomes necessary, patients can get a kidney transplant.

# 9

**❋ ❋ ❋**

# SCLERODERMA
# AND THE
# GASTROINTESTINAL
# TRACT

This information applies to people with systemic scleroderma, either limited or diffuse, and those with scleroderma sine sclerosis. It does not apply, or only rarely applies, to people with localized scleroderma (the morphea or linear type).

## *Background: How the GI Tract Works*

Almost everyone with systemic scleroderma (about 85 percent of cases) has some degree of GI (gastrointestinal) tract involvement, from mild to severe. The GI tract includes the esophagus, the stomach, the small bowel or intestine, the large bowel or colon, and the rectum (see Figure 1 on page 77). It is made up of a special kind of muscle called smooth muscle, which is different from the striated (skel-etal) muscles in the arms and legs. The main pathological process that happens in the GI tract in scleroderma is that the normal smooth muscle tissue is replaced by fibrotic scar tissue, a result of the fibroblasts' excessive production of collagen.

Smooth muscle is not under conscious control like skel-etal muscle, but is automatically controlled through a sys-tem of nerves called the autonomic nervous system. The purpose of the GI tract is to propel food and fluid in one direction from the mouth to the rectum, to absorb nutri-ents and to get rid of wastes. It begins with the swallowing mechanism in the upper throat, which forms the transition between voluntary chewing motion in the mouth, the semi-controlled motion of initiating swallowing, and the automatic motion of taking the swallowed material into the stomach. We all have had the sensation of chewing something and starting to swallow and then being able to stop swallowing and bring the food back up to the front of the mouth by clearing the throat or coughing. That is, we blow air up from the lungs to propel the food out of the back of the throat. Once the food is beyond this point in the back of the throat, however, it cannot be brought back up easily. After food is swallowed, the reflexes from the autonomic nervous system coordinate the contraction of the muscles so that food is propelled efficiently through the esophagus to the stomach. There is a special structure at the gastroe-sophageal (GE) junction (the place where the esophagus joins the stomach) called the lower esophageal sphincter. It pre-vents the stomach contents from going backward up the esophagus. This does not seem like much of a feat, since people usually eat sitting up and gravity alone would direct

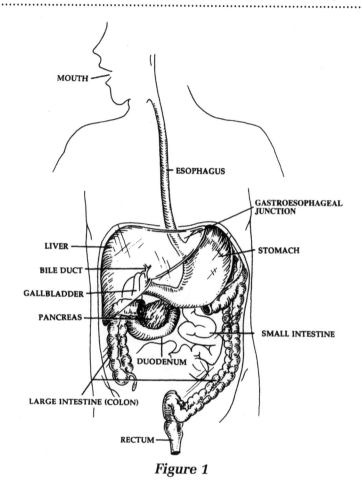

**MOUTH**

**ESOPHAGUS**

**GASTROESOPHAGEAL JUNCTION**

**LIVER**

**STOMACH**

**BILE DUCT**

**GALLBLADDER**

**PANCREAS**

**SMALL INTESTINE**

**DUODENUM**

**LARGE INTESTINE (COLON)**

**RECTUM**

*Figure 1*

food into the stomach. However, consider the situation of someone lying down and eating. If the muscles work normally, what is swallowed still gets to the stomach and stays there. As a matter of fact, if this system is working properly, people can stand on their heads and not have stomach acid travel up (or in this case down) the esophagus into the mouth.

The normally working esophagus, therefore, propels food and fluid down the esophagus, through the GE junction (one way only), and into the stomach, where it mixes with stomach acid, which starts to break down the food into smaller segments that can be absorbed. The stomach contents are emptied into the first part of the small bowel, called the duodenum, and pass by the common bile duct, which adds bile salts to break down fats, and also adds pancreatic enzymes to break down protein and carbohydrates. All of this mixture continues on down the length of the small bowel, where the lining cells that form the mucous membrane start to absorb all the good stuff (nutrients) and let pass all the indigestible stuff (roughage). The roughage gets dumped into the large bowel or colon, which is the first place in this process that involves bacteria. The gut, from the level of the stomach through the small intestine, is usually sterile, due to the action of the acid and the enzymes in the stomach juice and bile. This is pretty strong stuff and is capable of killing most bacteria and many viruses.

The large bowel does two things: It absorbs water, and it utilizes normally occurring bowel bacteria to break down the bile salts, which are reabsorbed and recycled. The rectum holds the fecal material (feces or stool, in medical terms) until it is released by the muscles of the anus, which are back under conscious control.

Now let us consider some pathological or disease conditions that change this smoothly functioning mechanism. First let us look at what happens with a common viral infection like the flu. As I mentioned above, many but not all viruses are killed by stomach acid and bile. Some viruses are not killed but pass through the GI tract without causing trouble. But there are particular viruses that are specially adapted to latch on to the cells of the mucosal lining (the lining of the

GI tract) and infect them, leading to viral gastroenteritis, sometimes called stomach flu. The body, in an attempt to get rid of the virus, speeds up the motion of the bowel (called peristalsis). This results in diarrhea, which gets rid of the material in the intestines. The body may even reverse the normal direction in the upper tract, vomiting material from the stomach and even, sometimes, from the duodenum. You may feel miserable, but the autonomic nervous system is doing what it is supposed to do under the circumstances, which is to get rid of the virus as soon as possible.

Another common problem in the general population is constipation. The most common cause of constipation in our society is lack of adequate fiber in the diet and not drinking enough water. Lack of exercise contributes as well. But in scleroderma, alternating diarrhea and constipation can occur from a different combination of circumstances.

### *Reflux*

Gastroesophageal reflux disease (GERD) is the most common GI problem associated with scleroderma. The primary symptom of reflux is heartburn. This is a painful, burning sensation felt near the bottom of the breastbone (the sternum). Since the stomach tends to lie on the left side of the upper abdomen, the burning frequently seems as though it is coming from the left side of the chest and can be mistaken for chest pain coming from the heart, hence the term "heartburn." The burning is actually caused by stomach acid flowing backward (reflux means "backward flow") into the esophagus. Whereas the lining cells of the stomach are especially suited to withstand stomach acid, the lining cells of the esophagus are not and can be damaged by persistent or recurring acid reflux.

How do you tell if a burning sensation near the breastbone is due to scleroderma or to normal heartburn, a common experience in the general population? There are some situations in which heartburn is so common it is considered normal. For example, during pregnancy, smooth muscle tissue relaxes, making the GE junction less tight, and the pregnant uterus also pushes against the stomach. Consequently, when a pregnant women bends over or lies down, she can experience heartburn. Additionally, the lower esophageal sphincter at the GE junction tends to weaken with age, so heartburn becomes more common as people get older. Being overweight with more fat in the midsection will also contribute to reflux. A hiatal hernia, in which part of the stomach extends into the chest through the diaphragm, will cause heartburn. Many people experience heartburn if they eat particularly spicy foods because the spices stimulate stomach acid production.

However, the reflux associated with scleroderma is different from the above situations in that it occurs on a daily basis, usually several times a day, regardless of the type of food eaten. This situation is a clear-cut change for the individual. Reflux or GERD associated with scleroderma is caused by the weakening of the muscles at the lower end of the esophagus, which normally prevent stomach acid from coming back up.

### Dysphagia

With continued acid reflux over time, scar tissue can build up and cause the swallowing passage to narrow. This narrowed area is called a stricture. Patients complain that they eat a small amount and the first few bites may be okay, but then something seems to get "caught." Sometimes they can force the food down by drinking water. Other times the only way they can relieve this feeling is to make themselves throw up. Many people will consciously or unconsciously change their diet so they don't eat large bites of meat or even large chunks of bread, or they always drink a lot of liquid as they eat and chew food thoroughly. Some people will change to an almost totally liquid diet to avoid this problem. I had one patient whose weight dropped to 90 pounds due to an esophageal stricture that caused her to switch to a liquid diet. After an esophageal dilatation (opening) with an instrument called an endoscope, she was able to eat normally and gained 40 pounds, returning to her usual weight.

Occasionally trouble swallowing (dysphagia) occurs even without formation of a stricture. Food seems to "hang up" in the esophagus. This occurs because there is ineffective peristalsis or muscle power to propel the food into the stomach. The muscles of the esophagus are replaced by scar tissue. Sitting upright to eat, eating slowly, chewing food thoroughly, and drinking fluid with the food are all good strategies to help with this. The way to determine if this is happening, or if there is an esophageal stricture, is to do a special X-ray called a cine esophagram. This is a procedure that uses a motion-picture camera to record the contractions of the esophageal smooth muscle as the patient swallows a drink containing barium. There is a distinctive pattern in the scleroderma-affected esophagus that differentiates it from a hiatal hernia and that helps to make the diagnosis. A stricture is readily seen with this X-ray as well. If the diagnosis of scleroderma is firm and the only reason to do the test is to see if a stricture is present, then a simple barium swallow will be adequate without the motion-picture part.

In addition to strictures, ulcers can occur in the esophagus from acid damage. These can make swallowing painful. Reflux of stomach acid can occur not just when eating, but at any time, especially on lying down. Small amounts of stomach acid can back up into the throat when people are sleeping and can be breathed into the larynx, causing damage to the vocal cords and a hoarse voice and/or sore throat in the morning. Stomach acid can sometimes be breathed into the lungs, contributing to lung irritation and lung fibrosis. Clearly there are many reasons to treat this condition.

Esophageal spasm (a sudden contraction or cramp in the esophagus) can occur due to a combination of many of these problems. This is a sudden and very painful condition resulting in severe chest pain and pressure. Most of my patients who have experienced this have gone to the emergency room, afraid that they were having a heart attack. Only after the doctors conclude from EKGs and blood tests that the heart is okay can they determine that the pain must have been coming from another source such as the esophagus.

Barrette's esophagus is a precancerous condition resulting from chronic inflammation of the lower part of the esophagus. As mentioned above, the cells that line the esophagus are not adapted to a highly acidic environment, as are the lining cells of the stomach. In some cases, the body responds to this chronic acid irritation by changing the cell type of the esophagus. Although these cellular changes are not a true cancer in the early stages, their presence means that there is an increased likelihood that cancer will develop. In this situation, annual endoscopy and biopsy are suggested. This involves examination of the esophagus and taking a sample of cells for a biopsy. Like most cancers, if detected early, treatment can lead to a cure.

Painful swallowing can be caused by an esophageal stricture or esophageal spasm, but for people on antibiotics, the possibility of a yeast infection of the esophagus (candida esophagitis) should be considered. The diagnosis is made by endoscopy. If present, the yeast infection can be cleared up with a special antifungal drug.

Occasionally scleroderma patients will have an infection in the stomach with a bacterium (*Helicobacter pylori*) that is the most common cause of ulcers in the general population. There is now a blood test to check for this infection. The point of getting the test is that if the infection is present, symptoms will improve with antibiotic treatment, though this will not eliminate the scleroderma-related scar tissue in the esophagus, stomach, or bowel.

### Treatments for Reflux

There are now excellent medications on the market to treat reflux. These are called proton pump inhibitors, which are frequently superior to the usual ulcer medications. Additionally, medicine that stimulates the action of smooth muscle (called prokinetic agents) can be used in conjunction with the proton pump inhibitors to treat reflux. Remember, the goal is not just to prevent the discomfort of heartburn, but also to avoid the development of esophageal ulcers, strictures, vocal-cord irritation, and possible lung fibrosis.

For the above reasons, even if they are on medication, patients should observe the following antireflux precautions:

1.  Don't eat within two hours of bedtime.
2.  Eat sitting up, eat slowly, and chew food carefully.
3.  Drink sips of water between bites and make sure each mouthful is fully swallowed before taking the next bite.
4.  Elevate the head of the bed at least four inches, using bricks or old phone books, for example. Do not simply elevate your head with a couple of pillows; you will slide off at night, and the angle of your head and body may make the reflux worse. There are special wedge pillows that start at the level of the low back and raise the head about four to six inches. This gradual slope is better than the use of two pillows.

The treatment for esophageal spasm is, surprisingly, the same as the treatment for angina (angina is true heart pain, caused by a decrease in blood supply to the heart muscle), and that is nitroglycerin tablets under the tongue. However, I recommend this only after the patient has had a thorough workup for heart disease and it is clear that the chest pain is not coming from the heart.

Although most people with scleroderma (about 85 percent) will have esophageal problems to some degree, not all will have severe problems. Many patients will have only mild reflux symptoms even after many years of scleroderma. It is impossible to accurately predict who will have bad problems and who will have only mild involvement. One of my goals in writing this book is to include all, or virtually all, of the possible problems that could develop, so that every scleroderma patient could find herself or himself in these pages. In over 20 years of caring for hundreds of patients, I have never yet seen one patient with all these complications.

### Problems of the Stomach and Small Bowel

The stomach can be involved in scleroderma in several ways: (1) the stomach is slow to empty, leading to a sense of feeling full after eating only a small amount, frequently accompanied by nausea, (2) erosions or ulcer formation occur as a result of acid buildup and sometimes as a consequence of medications, and (3) telangiectasias, or dilated blood vessels, that can bleed are present in the stomach. This last condition has been dubbed "watermelon stomach" due to the striped appearance of the dilated blood vessels as seen on endoscopy. This is also called GAVE for gastric antral vascular ectasia. The treatment for the first two conditions is the use of proton pump inhibitors or ulcer medicines coupled with the prokinetic agents mentioned above. The treatment for the third condition may include the use of female hormones, which have the unexpected effect of shrinking these blood vessels. In some cases the blood vessels can be treated with a laser through the endoscope. In severe cases surgical removal of part of the stomach may be required.

As the muscle of the small bowel becomes replaced by scar tissue, the bowel tends to slow down. The first symptom may be a sense of bloating after eating, a sign that food is slow to move along the GI tract. People may complain of increased gassiness. There may be cramping, which is caused by an unusually hard contraction of bowel muscle in an attempt to force material through. Pain in the bowel is usually caused by distention or expansion of one segment. Swallowed air or gas from bacterial digestion can get caught behind food material that gets "stuck" due to the slow transit. As this gas expands, it triggers the pain receptors.

Some people with constipation do well on a high-fiber diet, but others think that this worsens their gassiness. Foods such as beans, which are high gas producers, should be avoided. Exercise—for example, walking after meals—helps promote motion in the bowel. A stool softener containing sodium dodecyl sulfate can be helpful. (There are several brand names; talk to your pharmacist.) For the most part, laxatives should be avoided. These may help the problem in the short run but can make constipation worse in the long run. If you do use laxatives, consult your doctor and have a plan to minimize their use.

The preceding sections explain why people with scleroderma get constipated. But why does diarrhea happen?

As mentioned above in the section on how the normal GI tract works, the small bowel is normally free from bacteria. When the motion of the bowel is slowed, however, bacteria from the large bowel can spread backward into the small bowel, creating a situation called bacterial overgrowth. These bacteria then break down the bile acids that are needed for fat digestion; the result is that fats cannot be absorbed, causing diarrhea and weight loss. The process is called malabsorption. The diarrhea can go on for weeks or months and cause considerable loss of weight. One of my patients went from 240 pounds to 140 pounds over a 15-month period. This type of weight loss can result in vitamin deficiency, which in turn leads to many other problems.

The treatment for this kind of diarrhea is much different from that for the usual type of diarrhea, which comes with the flu or food poisoning. Most of the ordinary types of diarrhea will go away on their own after a few days. However, the diarrhea from bacterial overgrowth should be treated with a course of antibiotics; consult your doctor. For this problem it's best to take antibiotics for a short period of time, ten to fourteen days, followed by a period of a few weeks off medication, followed by another two weeks or so of treatment. Sometimes the diarrhea can be controlled after a few rounds of this type of therapy, and people can go for months or years without another treatment cycle. Occasionally people need to be on some form of antibiotics almost continuously. Another strategy involves finding out whether particular foods make the problem worse. Some people find that dairy foods will exacerbate the diarrhea. In those cases, avoidance of milk, ice cream, and cheese is a good idea. Since these foods are an excellent source of calcium, I do not recommend their avoidance to everyone. I suggest a trial-and-error system to see what works for you.

This is another situation in which the prokinetic agents are used. These medications can be very helpful in improving the motion of the bowel muscle that is left, but once the fibrosis reaches a severe level (which, fortunately, happens only in rare cases), there is not enough muscle left to stimulate. In addition to pills, there is an injectable medication called somatostatin that can be helpful in very severe cases.

If the bowel problem doesn't respond to these approaches, there are two options. The first is tube feeding with an elemental diet, which is a solution of ready-to-absorb protein, fats, and carbohydrates with added vitamins and minerals. It tastes truly horrible and is meant to be taken through a tube directly into the stomach or small bowel. However, in individuals whose small bowel is not capable of handling even this fluid, the only alternative is intravenous feeding using an indwelling IV line, usually inserted into the large vein under the collarbone. The special IV lines are meant to stay for months at a time, and the IV solution can be hooked up for several hours usually at night. Difficulties arise in that all the connections must be kept sterile, and the IV tube can get clotted off, requiring a replacement. Over the past 20 years I have had only a handful of patients (out of more than 1,000) who have required intravenous feedings because their GI tract simply would not move food along.

### The Large Bowel

Involvement of the large bowel usually manifests as constipation. On testing with a barium enema, large outpouchings called diverticuli can be seen. These seldom if ever cause diverticulitis, which is an inflammation of a smaller type of outpouching that tends to occur in many people as they get older. The treatment for this type of constipation is the same as for constipation of the usual variety, that is, stool softeners on a regular basis, a diet with adequate fiber (avoiding high-fiber foods that are high gas producers), exercise such as a walking program, and the cautious and only occasional use of laxatives.

Another cause of constipation is hypothyroidism, or an underactive thyroid. This is more common in scleroderma patients than in the general population, so a blood test for thyroid function should be done to consider this possibility. If the thyroid is not functioning properly, supplemental thyroid hormone should be taken. This is available in pill form.

### Anemia from Bleeding in the GI Tract

Anemia, or low hemoglobin in the blood, can occur in scleroderma patients as a direct result of the scleroderma itself, in which case it is called *anemia of chronic disease*, or as a result of blood loss through the GI tract. This is most frequently caused by bleeding from esophagitis or esophageal ulcers, from stomach ulcers, or from the dilated blood vessels in "watermelon stomach." The best approach is to identify the source of the bleeding with one of the tests mentioned at the end of this chapter and direct treatment toward that particular problem. Sometimes transfusions are necessary if the anemia becomes severe. Iron supplements can help if the anemia is due to blood loss and not to the anemia of chronic disease. However, iron tends to be hard on the digestive tract and can cause nausea, vomiting, abdominal cramping, and diarrhea on its own

### Coordinating Your Care

So who is your doctor under these circumstances—your rheumatologist or your gastroenterologist? Since scleroderma can affect many organs and since no one doctor can do all the procedures you may require, you will end up with a series of doctors. Sometimes one doctor will tell you one thing and another will tell you the opposite. What you need is a "quarterback," one person to do the coordinating, to know all the medications you are on, and to make sure they are not in conflict. This is usually the rheumatologist, but you need to decide along with your doctor who this will be. Managed-care plans can sometimes make it difficult to get referrals, but you have to get in the driver's seat. You (yes, you) have to make sure that reports are sent from one doctor to the next. It may be necessary for you to ask for a copy for your own personal records and then make sure that copies are distributed to all your doctors. It is okay to request this, and you don't have to be able to understand what the reports say.

* * *

At right is a summary of the tests that are available and frequently used in scleroderma. I certainly do not use all these tests in all patients with GI problems. Sometimes the situation is so clear that I feel I don't need to do any testing. As a general rule of thumb, I order tests when the clinical situation is not clear-cut or when another disease or condition can be present that would require a different therapeutic approach.

### *Summary of GI Tests:*

**Barium swallow:** an X ray test that can determine if a stricture is present in the esophagus or if there is a hiatal hernia; this requires swallowing a liquid with barium dissolved in it (barium shows up white on an X ray)

**Cine esophagram:** an X ray test similar to the barium swallow that takes an X ray movie of the motion of the espophagus; this can determine if there is decreased motion of the esophageal muscles of the type seen in scleroderma

**Upper GI series:** a barium swallow that follows the barium through the stomach into the small bowel; it can also pick up some stomach ulcers or tumors

**Transit study:** the measurement of the time it takes for material to go from the stomach through the bowel

**Hydrogen breath study:** a test to determine how much of a sample meal is absorbed; this can determine if there are bacteria in the small bowel, so this is a test for malabsorption

**Upper endoscopy:** a test in which a tube (endoscope) is passed through the mouth into the esophagus and stomach so that the doctor can see the lining of the esophagus and stomach, and inflammation, ulcers, enlarged blood vessels, bleeding sites, and tumors can be directly visualized. A biopsy to remove a tiny piece of tissue can be taken through the endoscope to be examined under the microscope. If a stricture is present, a balloon can be inflated and the area of stricture enlarged or dilated.

This is a very useful procedure for the kinds of problems that scleroderma patients typically have. One difficulty is that it may be hard to pass the endoscope through the mouth in some scleroderma patients due to inability to open the mouth very far. To get around this problem, a pediatric (child-sized) endoscope can be used.

**Lower endoscopy** or **colonscopy:** a test in which a tube (colonscope) is passed through the anus into the rectum and large bowel; this is useful in detecting cancer, polyps, or sources of bleeding in the colon

**Sigmoidoscopy:** a test in which a tube is passed through the anus only as far as the rectum and part of the colon

### Treatment Summary

*For reflux:* proton pump inhibitor or other ulcer medicine, frequently with a prokinetic agent; reflux precautions include avoiding eating near bedtime, elevating the head of bed, and so on

*For decreased motion (decreased peristalsis):* prokinetic agent

*For bacterial overgrowth and malabsorption:* antibiotic or a combination of antibiotics

*For constipation:* a stool softener on a regular basis, daily or every other day, plus a diet with adequate fiber and a walking exercise program

*For watermelon stomach:* female hormones (*in male patients only*), endoscopic cauterization, or removal of part of the stomach

# 10
✳ ✳ ✳

# SCLERODERMA
# AND THE LUNGS

Before I begin to discuss how scleroderma can affect the lungs, it is helpful to describe normal lung structure and function. The purpose of the lungs is pretty simple: to extract oxygen from the air we breathe (normal room air is 21 percent oxygen) and to get rid of carbon dioxide ($CO_2$), which is a byproduct of metabolism, the process of converting food products to energy. To do this, the lungs consist of thousands of tiny air sacs (one air sac is an *alveolus*, more than one are called *alveoli*), which are arranged around breathing tubes like grapes on a stalk. Air is brought in through the nose and mouth, pulled into the main breathing tube through the voice box, or larynx, and into the trachea, or windpipe (see Figure 2). This divides into the right and left main-stem bronchi, large tubes that in turn branch into smaller and smaller air tubes until they reach the smallest

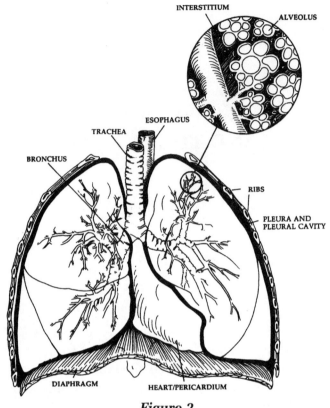

INTERSTITIUM

ALVEOLUS

ESOPHAGUS

TRACHEA

BRONCHUS

RIBS

PLEURA AND
PLEURAL CAVITY

DIAPHRAGM

HEART/PERICARDIUM

*Figure 2*

tubes, called *bronchioles*, which have clusters of alveoli around them. The exchange of oxygen for carbon dioxide occurs only in the alveoli. Each alveolus has a very thin lining or wall composed of a mucous membrane cell on the inside, where the air is, and a capillary (the smallest type of blood vessel) on the outside. Separating the lining cell and the capillary is a very thin structure called a basement membrane, which is made up of collagen.

Blood returning to the heart through the veins passes through the tiny alveolar capillaries one red cell at a time. Since this is venous blood, the red cell has already lost its oxygen, having given it up to tissues. Oxygen diffuses or passes from the air you breathe into the alveolus across the thin basement membrane into the capillary blood, gets picked up by the hemoglobin in the red cell—hemoglobin is a wonderful molecule with a strong affinity for oxygen; it is also what makes red blood cells red—and gets carried off to the heart for another pass around the circulatory system. As oxygen is diffusing in, carbon dioxide, which is dissolved in the blood serum, passes out of the blood into the air into the alveolus, because the concentration of carbon dioxide in air is much less than in venous blood.

What goes wrong in scleroderma? The basement membrane, between the mucous membrane lining cell and the capillary, is composed of collagen, and scleroderma causes additional collagen to be deposited in this membrane, making it thicker than normal and making it harder and harder for the oxygen to get through into the capillaries. The cell responsible for making this collagen is the pulmonary fibroblast, which resides, along with the mucous membrane lining cell, in the alveolus. Ordinarily the fibroblast doesn't make much collagen; it exists to repair damage from infections, such as pneumonia, or irritation, such as breathing in tiny particles of sand (as, for example, in coal miner's lung disease, or black lung).

What stimulates the fibroblast to make more collagen in scleroderma? There is no apparent infection and no known irritant, so what is going on? We don't know what the initial trigger is, but we do know that there is a cascade of factors coming from activated immune cells and/or damaged blood vessel lining cells, all of which work to activate the fibroblasts.

*Alveolitis* is the term used to describe the pathological or diseased lung process in scleroderma. This refers to the fact that there is an inflammation in the small air sacs, leading to fibrosis. Sometimes this process goes on slowly and quietly, causing no symptoms until there has been a lot of lung damage. In the early stages, a chest X-ray can be normal, but a high-resolution CAT scan of the lungs will be abnormal. Pulmonary function tests are very sensitive in picking up changes in lung function, but they will not distinguish between new fibrosis and old, inactive fibrosis.

*Pulmonary fibrosis* is the term used to describe the scar-tissue buildup in the lungs. Pulmonary fibrosis can be caused by conditions other than scleroderma. These include an inherited form of fibrosis (seen in multiple family members), a reaction to stone dust (seen in miners and sandblasters), or a reaction to some forms of lung inflammation, called adult respiratory distress syndrome (ARDS). These are all fairly unusual occurrences, so the appearance of pulmonary fibrosis on a chest X-ray or the development of a restrictive pattern on pulmonary function tests in a scleroderma patient usually means that the fibrosis is due to scleroderma-related lung involvement.

### Symptoms

The two major symptoms of pulmonary involvement in scleroderma are coughing and shortness of breath. The cough is usually dry, that is, there is little or no sputum or mucus production. There are several reasons why people can have a chronic or recurrent cough, and there are many reasons for people to be short of breath, so it is necessary to consider all the possibilities before alveolitis can be blamed.

The most common cause of cough in my scleroderma patients is seasonal allergies, totally unrelated to their scleroderma but very much related to the climate. Every spring and every fall, these patients get a feeling of fullness in the nasal passages and sinuses, and they experience postnasal drip, hoarseness, cough, and so on. This also occurs in my lupus and arthritis patients. The point of this is that not every cough in a scleroderma patient is due to scleroderma-related lung disease. But if a cough is persistent, lasting more than six weeks, and is not associated with other signs of allergies, flu, or colds, then a diagnosis of alveolitis should be considered.

The first step in the workup is usually pulmonary function tests (PFTs), including a diffusion capacity, which measures the efficiency of gas exchange across the pulmonary membrane. In this test, people breathe into a machine that measures airflow and lung volumes. There are three general patterns of lung abnormalities: asthma, emphysema, and fibrosis. One of the problems in interpreting this test is that in the early stages of scleroderma-related alveolitis there may be enough inflammation to evoke a cough response, but there is not yet enough fibrosis to make the test results very abnormal. Another complicating factor is lung damage due to smoking. Such damage will be picked up on the PFTs, confusing the picture and making the test results more difficult to interpret. As mentioned above, in the early stages the chest X-ray is frequently normal. If this is the case, then a high-resolution CAT scan of the chest should be done to try to pick up the "ground glass" appearance of alveolitis in the lung bases. If this is present, then the diagnosis is firm.

In many situations the picture is not clear-cut, and your doctor may be concerned that there is an underlying infection responsible for the cough. If this is the case, the only way to determine the type of infection is by doing a biopsy that involves getting a small piece of lung tissue. A biopsy can be done with a bronchoscope, a procedure in which a tube is passed into the lungs and the biopsy taken through the tube. At the time of this procedure, broncho-alveolar lavage (BAL) can also be done through the bronchoscope. In BAL, fluid is first introduced into one area of the lung and then removed by suction. In the removed fluid there are inflammatory cells washed out from the alveoli. These cells can then be analyzed both for the typical pattern of scleroderma and for various infections.

Alternatively, an open biopsy can be done. This is a surgical procedure in which an incision is made in the side of the chest and a piece of lung removed. This yields a larger piece of lung tissue and a better sample. However, this is a surgical procedure that requires general anesthesia and involves a recovery procedure of several days, whereas bronchoscopy can usually be done as an outpatient with "light" sedation.

The bottom line for all of this is that the diagnosis can be unclear. It is essential to make the correct diagnosis, since the treatment of alveolitis is very different from the treatment of an underlying infection and, in fact, might worsen an infection. One or more of these tests may need to be done in order for the diagnosis to be made with certainty. Treatment will be outlined later in this chapter.

Shortness of breath is the other main symptom of scleroderma lung involvement. However, like the development of a cough, it is not specific for alveolitis or fibrosis and can be caused by a number of other things. Shortness of breath, from whatever cause, usually is first noticed with exertion. People complain that they get more winded going up a flight of stairs than they used to. Or they may notice that whereas they used to be able to walk several blocks with ease, now they can walk only one block or have to slow their pace to go more than one block due to shortness of breath. One patient told me that the street in front of his house seemed to have gotten longer.

The main causes of shortness of breath in scleroderma patients are the following: (1) pulmonary fibrosis, (2) deconditioning (being out of shape), (3) a heart problem, (4) muscle weakness due to inflammation (polymyositis) or an underactive thyroid, (5) anemia, or a low red cell count, and (6) pulmonary hypertension. How is all of this sorted out? The chest X-ray and pulmonary function tests (PFTs) are helpful, especially if they were done in the previous year or so for comparison. An echocardiogram (ultrasound of the heart) can be very helpful to evaluate heart function and also to test for pulmonary hypertension. Blood tests will help to determine whether there is muscle inflammation, a thyroid problem, or anemia. If the results of all these tests are normal, then the culprit is deconditioning, which is to say that you are out of shape, and the approach is one of physical therapy and exercise.

What if the news is not that good and the diagnosis is alveolitis? What are the available treatment options? Before that question can be answered, I need to distinguish between active inflammation (alveolitis) and established pulmonary fibrosis. Alveolitis should be treated; nonprogressive fibrosis may not need to be.

## *Treatment of Alveolitis*

It is not clear what the best treatment of scleroderma alveolitis should be. The National Institutes of Health (NIH) is currently conducting a multicenter trial of a medicine called cyclophosphamide (Cytoxan, a form of chemotherapy), in early alveolitis in scleroderma lung disease. The results of this multicenter trial should be known in mid-2005. In the meantime, many physicians use this medication with or without prednisone to see if it helps. There is some variation among scleroderma specialists in treatment regimens, particularly in the dose of prednisone and in whether the cyclophosphamide is given as a single intravenous dose on a monthly basis for six to twelve months or as daily pills for the same length of time. The multicenter trial will answer some of these questions. Other medications that are sometimes used include azathioprine (Imuran) or mycophenolate mofetil (Cellcept) but the evidence to support the use of these drugs in scleroderma is somewhat weak.

The side effects of prednisone (also known as cortisone or glucocorticoid medication) are multiple and can be severe, depending on the dose and the individual's particular reaction. The potential side effects of cyclophosphamide are also serious. This is one of the reasons that physicians like to be very sure about the diagnosis before they recommend this treatment. I will not go into all the potential side effects of these medications here, since I think that this is best discussed between the patient and the doctor on a one-to-one basis. In this situation, the patient has to consider what the alternative to treatment is. If no treatment is given, alveolitis will likely worsen and result in pulmonary fibrosis. In some cases, this is progressive over a course of several years and results in pulmonary failure.

### Treatment of Nonprogressive Pulmonary Fibrosis

Some individuals have no cough and no shortness of breath, but on physical examination have some abnormal sounds (*rales*) when the doctor listens to the lung bases (the bottom of the lungs at the back). A chest X-ray may show some scar tissue at the bases, and the PFTs can show a restrictive pattern characteristic of scleroderma lung disease. A high-resolution CAT scan of the chest may only show the scar tissue and not demonstrate the "ground glass" appearance of inflammation (active alveolitis). What should be done in this instance? Should prednisone and chemotherapy be given in an attempt to slow down or stop this from getting worse?

The answer depends on the rate of development of the fibrosis. If it is clear that the results of the PFTs have worsened recently and are continuing to worsen, then treatment should be considered. However, I also believe there is time to observe and get a sense of the rapidity of the worsening, especially if there are no recent pulmonary tests that can be used for comparison. In the absence of symptoms (that is, no cough and no shortness of breath), it is reasonable to wait three to six months and repeat the PFTs. If they are not changing over time, then there is no need to treat. This may be the case when the lung fibrosis is a reaction to reflux, that is, a reaction to small amounts of stomach acid being breathed into the lungs at night. If so, I would recommend antireflux precautions and heartburn medication.

If, however, there is a slow and gradual decline in the pulmonary function test values, then I think it is very important to treat the problem. As mentioned, the study to determine if Cytoxan is helpful is currently underway, and there is no strong evidence that other medications are effective.

In very advanced cases, a lung transplant can be considered. However, the availability of lungs for transplant is low, and there is concern that fibrosis may occur in the new transplanted lung. Actually, this seldom happens due to the use of antirejection drugs that suppress the immune system. However, all these factors have kept transplantation from being a viable option for many scleroderma patients.

### *Pulmonary Hypertension*

Isolated pulmonary hypertension (high blood pressure in the lungs) is a different type of complication that occurs in about 15 to 25 percent of scleroderma patients. It can occur with very normal, or even low, systemic blood pressure as measured in the arm. In order to understand this, it is necessary once again to review some anatomy regarding the circulation of blood. Blood leaves the left side of the heart, goes into the arteries, and supplies oxygen to the body. In the process it picks up carbon dioxide and returns via the veins to the right side of the heart. The right side of the heart then pumps it into the lungs through the pulmonary artery. In the lungs, the venous blood gets rid of the carbon dioxide, picks up oxygen, and goes to the left side of the heart to be pumped out to the body again as arterial blood.

Arterial blood is oxygenated and appears bright red; venous blood has lost most of its oxygen and appears dark red or bluish. Arterial blood is under higher pressure than venous blood, so if you puncture an artery, it squirts with every heartbeat. If you puncture a vein, it just oozes blood. Most arteries are buried deeper than veins, to protect them. When you get blood drawn, the technician pokes a vein. However, to get arterial blood gases, or ABGs, for an accurate measurement of the total oxygen in the blood, an artery has to be punctured, and pressure has to be applied for several minutes afterward to stop the bleeding. Rather than get blood gases, I frequently order an oxygen saturation measurement by ear oximetry, which can be done without a needle stick. The information obtained is somewhat different from that given by the ABGs, but the oximetry can be done easily before and after exercise, which is a valuable comparison in individuals who complain about shortness of breath on exertion.

Back to pulmonary hypertension. The pressure in the pulmonary artery needs to be just high enough to push the blood through the lungs. This requires less pressure than that needed to push the blood through the rest of the body. There are two things that can raise pulmonary pressure. One is the loss of volume capacity of the lung vessels. This means that with every heartbeat, the right ventricle (the pumping chamber on the right side) has to try to push the same volume of blood into a smaller volume of space, causing a rise in pressure. This loss of volume capacity happens in extensive pulmonary fibrosis because the capillaries end up "choked off" and can no longer carry as much blood.

Another example of loss of volume capacity is when a lung is surgically removed, for example in lung cancer surgery.

However, there is a particular kind of pulmonary hypertension that occurs in the absence of extensive fibrosis and for no apparent reason. This is referred to as isolated pulmonary hypertension and results from a loss of elasticity of the pulmonary artery that becomes narrowed. The right ventricle is trying to pump the same volume of blood into a smaller-diameter tube, so the pressure has to go up. An analogy is a garden hose with an adjustable nozzle. With the nozzle wide open, the pressure is pretty low. As you adjust the nozzle down to a smaller opening, the pressure becomes higher.

What causes this narrowing of the pulmonary artery? And what are the consequences of the higher pressure? I'll answer the second question first. The pumping chamber of the right side of the heart is not made to generate a lot of force. At first it can accommodate a small reduction in the lungs' volume capacity, but as the volume capacity falls, the heart cannot generate enough force to push all of the blood it receives into the lungs. So fluid will back up in the venous system, causing liver congestion and swelling in the lower extremities. This is known as right-sided heart failure.

The answer to the first question of what causes the narrowing is harder to explain. The muscle layer of the pulmonary arteries get larger, and the inside lining of the artery also gets thicker. The stimulus for all this is not clear.

In terms of diagnosing isolated pulmonary hypertension in scleroderma patients, the best test is an echocardiogram with special attention to the right side of the heart. If this clearly shows that the structures and pressure on the right side of the heart are normal, then it is unlikely that a significant degree of pulmonary hypertension is present. If the results are abnormal or difficult to interpret, a right heart catheterization should be done to more precisely measure the right-sided pressures. This is different from a left-heart catheterization that is usually done to evaluate coronary arteries and the risk of a heart attack.

In any event, what can be done about this? There are several approaches to treatment. Giving oxygen at night helps, since oxygen serves to relax the smooth muscle of the pulmonary artery. Unfortunately, most blood pressure medicines that work quite nicely for systemic hypertension (the more common type of hypertension, measured by taking the arm blood pressure) have little effect on pressure in the pulmonary circulation. The blood thinner warfarin (Coumadin) is frequently given to prevent blood clots from forming in the narrowed blood vessels.

In addition to these measures, there are now three types of medication that are approved for the treatment of pulmonary arterial hypertension (PAH) in the United States. The first of these is epoprostanil (Flolan), which is given as a continuous IV infusion. An indwelling plastic tube is inserted into the large vein under the collarbone and attached to a small pump containing the medicine. The pump is carried as a waist pack or a shoulder pack. The medication has to be given 24 hours a day for the rest of a person's life —or until a better medicine comes along. This may seem like an extreme treatment, but it has been life saving for many individuals. Some of my patients who had previously been wheelchair bound and on oxygen 24 hours a day due to PAH, have been able to resume near-normal activities and go off the oxygen at least during the day.

The second medicine to be approved is treprostinil (Remodulin). This works in a similar fashion similar as Flolan but is given as a constant or continuous infusion through a small needle under the skin (subcutaneously) that is attached to a portable pump. This avoids the need for an indwelling IV line but has some problems of its own. The way that both Flolan and Remodulin work is by opening up or dilating blood vessels. When Remodulin is given under the skin, it causes the small vessels of the skin to dilate causing redness, soreness and sometimes itching at the site of the injection. Usually other medications like anti-inflammatory drugs or pain medication must be given as well to counteract these effects.

The third new medicine for PAH is bosentan (Tracleer). This is a pill that is given twice a day. Although a pill is a lot easier to take than an infusion, it appears to be less effective than the infused medicines, so patients with more severe PAH are usually started on one of the infusions. Over time it may be possible to transition to the pill. Those with milder PAH can start on the pill and may never need to go on to the other drugs. Various combinations of these medicines are now in clinical trials, as well as new medications. For those on Tracleer, a blood test that measures liver function has to be done on a monthly basis because about 10 percent of people will develop liver abnormalities. This will go back to normal once the medication is stopped.

As part of the studies that were done to prove safety and effectiveness in pulmonary hypertension, it was noted that patients who also had finger ulcers seemed to do better while on these medications. This has led to a new study to look at the effect of Tracleer on healing and preventing finger ulcers. There is also a study to determine if Tracleer can improve the lung inflammation (alveolitis) due to scleroderma. Results of these trials should be known in early 2005.

Based on the success of these medicines, new drugs are being developed for PAH and for finger ulcers. One of these is an "old" drug known as sildenafil or Viagra. Although this usually gets a laugh from my mostly female scleroderma patients, there is some evidence that it can be helpful. Studies to answer this question are ongoing. In addition, new drugs that have similar mechanisms of action as the ones mentioned in this chapter are in various stages of development by pharmaceutical companies. From the point of view of the treating physician as well as from the point of view of the affected patient, this is good news. Never before in my more than 20 years of treating and studying scleroderma have there been such an interest and so many studies. Some of these trials will be negative, that is, the anticipated effect will not occur. But the fact that trials of three different medications have been positive is grounds for optimism. There are now more clinical trials in scleroderma than ever before. As someone who treats scleroderma patients and who also conducts these studies, this is good news indeed.

Should you take part in a clinical study? There are several reasons to do so, but you really need to know what you are getting yourself in for. There are several questions you need to ask yourself. Are you willing to accept the risk that you may get a placebo (a dummy medication)? Most of the studies in scleroderma, as well as other diseases, compare the effects of the new medication to that of a placebo or dummy pill. The new medicine may not be helpful and, in fact, may have some unpleasant or dangerous side effects, so being on the "real" medicine may not be the best thing.

Also, most studies are "randomized." This means that you do not get to choose to be in the real medicine group versus the placebo group. You are assigned to the group by chance, like with a flip of a coin. In addition, most studies are "double-blinded." This means that neither you nor the study physician know which group you are in. Both the real medicine and the placebo look alike so you cannot tell by looking at the pill which one it is. Because of these issues, most clinical trials will permit patients to go on the real medicine at the end of the study if they were on placebo, or to stay on the real medicine if that was the group they had been assigned to, as long as the study proved that it was safe and effective. The company that conducted the trial usually provides the medicine free of charge at least until the FDA (Food and Drug Administration) officially approves it.

Some people think that just because a drug company sponsors a clinical trial that the trial will always show the medicine to be safe and effective. I know (and my patients know) by firsthand experience that this is not always the case. I have been involved in several drug-company-sponsored studies that were "negative," that is we proved conclusively that the medicine did *not* work. This is also one of the reasons I am so excited about the new drugs for PAH, and why I am so hopeful that we can find safe and effective treatments for other aspects of scleroderma as well.

In terms of safety in drug trials, there are several safeguards that must be in place before a study can be conducted in human subjects. First of all, every study has to be reviewed by an Institutional Review Board (IRB) for the protection of human subjects. All medical schools and hospitals must have an IRB if they want to participate in research. The people who serve on this panel include physicians, scientists, nurses, ethicists, and members of the community. This panel determines if a study is ethical, and if it is likely to get results that will benefit patients. This group also reviews the progress of studies at least annually to make sure that they are being conducted the way they should be. In addition to this, treatment trials must have a separate Drug Safety and Monitoring Board who review all adverse events and who have the authority to stop a study if they feel that the risks exceed the benefits. All study records are monitored and there are penalties for not following the guidelines, up to and including losing the privilege to conduct studies as well as losing all grant funding. I have seen this system from both sides—as an investigator applying for approval to start a trial, and as a reviewer of trials (an investigator is not allowed to review his/her own study)—and I know that at least for the most part, the system works.

All patients who participate in a study must first sign a consent form that explains the purpose of the study, lists all the tests and visits that are required, and outlines the potential risks and benefits. This can be a pretty daunting process.

Even if you want to be in a study, you may not qualify. Every study has a list of inclusion and exclusion criteria that define who may be enrolled. Some studies are only meant for newly diagnosed patients, others are looking for patients with active lung disease or new finger ulcers. Most of the time, people are required to have fairly normal kidney and lung function to be considered candidates. It is not uncommon for me to screen three times as many patients as I actually enroll in a study due to these constraints.

Having read all of this, you may wonder why anyone would agree to take part. The answer varies with the individual. Some people have a sincere desire to help medical science; others are willing to take risks in order to get a new medication that may not be available to the general public for a few years. One of my patients called herself a "study veteran." She knew that her condition would be monitored more closely in a study setting and she felt comfortable with taking a risk. Although we don't pay people to be in a study, we at least provide free parking, occasionally a free lunch in the hospital cafeteria if the testing takes a long time (this may not be considered a real benefit), and a nice study nurse who calls periodically to check on people.

I also know people who have declined to be in studies because they were too anxious, both fearing they would be on placebo and therefore not getting treatment, and also fearing that they would be on the real medicine that might cause some bad side effect. The decision is a personal one and should not be influenced by the desire to please the doctor. I tell my patients that I won't be mad if they decline, that I will still see them as usual, and it is really "okay."

## Summary of Treatment for
### Alveolitis/Pulmonary Fibrosis

1. Stop smoking! Although scleroderma-related lung disease is different from that caused by tobacco, smoking will only make the lung process worse and will also make Raynaud's phenomenon worse.

2. Use measures to prevent gastroesophageal reflux (GERD): elevate the head of the bed, no eating within two hours of bedtime, take medication to treat heartburn, and so on (see Chapter 6).

3. If alveolitis or progressive pulmonary fibrosis is present, an immunosuppressive medication with or without prednisone should be used.

4. If nonprogressive pulmonary fibrosis is present, observe closely with periodic pulmonary function tests.

5. If severe fibrosis is present, home oxygen therapy may be needed.

6. In severe cases a lung transplant may be necessary.

## Summary of Treatment for
### Isolated Pulmonary Hypertension

1. Oxygen treatment at night, and occasionally during the day with activity.

2. Medication includes pills and/or injections or infusions of dilating agents.

# 11

✳ ✳ ✳

# SCLERODERMA
# AND THE HEART

Scleroderma can affect the heart in several ways. In some cases, heart rhythm can be affected. This is demonstrated by a slow or irregular heartbeat or by an abnormality that is seen only on an electrocardiogram (EKG or ECG). In these cases, the approach to treatment involves either medication to help keep the heartbeat regular or a pacemaker to override the natural electrical system that controls the heartbeat.

Heart rhythm is controlled by an electrical conduction system comprised of specialized cells that generate an electrical current to stimulate the heart muscle to contract in a smooth and regular way. There is a complex system of reflexes that tells the heart to speed up (as with exercise) or to slow down (as with rest), but there is only one electrical system that sends signals to both sides of the heart so that all four chambers contract or pump in a synchronized fashion. The problem that occurs in some cases of scleroderma is that scar tissue (the same culprit we have discussed in the previous chapters) is deposited in the path of the electrical current, so the current is interrupted or blocked. This can be partial or a complete block depending on exactly where it is and how much scar tissue is present. Sometimes the irregular heartbeat is noticed by the patient and sometimes not. It is important to get an EKG to determine exactly what type of problem exists. If no irregularity is picked up on the EKG, then a portable Holter monitor can be given to the patient, which records the EKG for an entire day. This test can pick up heart irregularities that occur only occasionally and are not captured during the short period of time that the EKG is recorded in the doctor's office.

Normal heart rhythm is called normal *sinus rhythm*, since the source of the electrical current comes from a structure in the heart called the *sinus node*. Changes from normal rhythms are called *arrhythmias*. There are different terms to describe the dozen or so possible different types of arrhythmias. There is a conduction abnormality called a *right bundle branch block*, which means that the electrical signal to the right side of the heart is impaired, and (as you would expect) there is a condition known as a *left bundle branch block*, affecting the left side; then there is a *complete heart block*. The complete heart block is not as lethal as it sounds, since there is a backup system that permits the heart to beat at a very slow rate (35–40 beats per minute, as opposed to the usual resting heart rate of 60–90 beats per minute) in the absence of sinus node activity. This is not a good situation for the long term, however, and a pacemaker is usually used in the case of complete heart block. There are several other types of cardiac arrhythmias that can happen, some of which make the heat beat too fast rather than too slowly. Some of these arrhythmias need to be treated with either medication or a pacemaker, while others do not.

There are conditions other than scleroderma that can cause conduction problems and arrhythmias. The most common of these conditions is coronary artery disease caused by cholesterol buildup; this is the main cause of heart attacks. Just because someone has scleroderma doesn't mean that they cannot get "regular" heart problems. Because of this, a cardiac catheterization may need to be done. If the diagnosis is usual coronary artery disease, then bypass surgery may be helpful in order to prevent a heart attack.

Another way that scleroderma can affect the heart happens when scar tissue is deposited throughout the heart muscle, not just limited to the conduction system, making it a less effective pump. In this case, medication such as digitalis can be helpful. Since there are other reasons why someone can have this type of problem, tests such as an echocardiogram as well as an EKG and possibly a stress test and a cardiac catheterization may need to be done to get a good picture of what is going on in a particular case and what is the best approach to treatment.

The third way that scleroderma can affect the heart is by causing inflammation in the outside membrane of the heart, which is called *pericarditis*. The pericardium is a sac that surrounds the heart. When the sac becomes inflamed, fluid accumulates. Sometimes this causes symptoms such as chest pain or shortness of breath, and sometimes it is discovered accidentally by your doctor during a visit for something else. Again, the way to make the diagnosis is by an echocardiogram. If there is a small

amount of fluid that does not compress the heart and therefore does not interfere with heart function, medication can
be used to treat the inflammation. Typically these medications are either steroids, such as prednisone, or nonsteroidal anti-inflammatory drugs (NSAIDs), such as arthritis
medications. If the amount of fluid is very small and there
are no symptoms, it is okay to do nothing and to watch the
situation. If, on the other hand, the fluid volume is quite
large and pressing against the heart, compromising the ability of the heart to fill, then a surgical procedure called a
pericardial window may need to be done. This permits the
fluid to drain out into the lung cavity, where there is more
space to accommodate it. Following this, the medication
mentioned above can be given to resolve the inflammation
over a period of a few weeks. The excess fluid eventually
gets reabsorbed back into the bloodstream. Pericarditis is a
temporary phenomenon. Although it may recur months or
years later, it will resolve again after treatment.

Pulmonary artery hypertension (PAH) is a blood-vessel
problem, not really a heart problem and is discussed in
more detail in chapter 10. Since PAH usually causes shortness of breath with activity, patients are frequently sent to
a lung specialist for evaluation rather than a cardiologist.
This is one of many situations in scleroderma when you
need a team of doctors (rheumatologist, pulmonologist, and
cardiologist) who can work together.

## Summary of Heart Involvement

1. Arrythmias are problems with heart rhythm that can be treated with medication or a pacemaker.

2. Heart failure is the inability of the heart to pump out as much blood as it receives; this is due to a problem with heart muscle function that is usually treated with medication.

3. Pericarditis is an inflammation of the sac that surrounds the heart and is treated either with medication or with a surgical procedure called placement of a pericardial window.

## Summary of Tests

1. *EKG:* an electrocardiogram, the heart tracing done in a doctor's office that measures heart rate and rhythm

2. *Holter monitor:* a portable EKG monitor usually worn for twenty-four hours to pick up heart rhythm irregularities that may be present only occasionally and that were not picked up by the usual EKG

3. *Echocardiogram:* an ultrasound test of the heart that measures heart function: how well the chambers of the heart are pumping, how well the heart valves are working, and if there is any excess fluid in the sac around the heart

4. *Cardiac catheterization:* a test in which a plastic tube is inserted into a large blood vessel, usually in the groin or in the arm, and threaded into the heart. Contrast material, or IV "dye," is injected into the heart or into the coronary arteries that supply blood to the heart muscle

to determine if any vessels are blocked by cholesterol plaques. This procedure can also measure pressures in the heart and in the pulmonary artery to determine if pulmonary hypertension is present.

5. *Cardiac stress test:* a test that determines if the heart is getting an adequate blood supply during exercise. Sometimes the heart will appear normal at rest, and it is only with stress that an abnormality can be demonstrated.

6. *Heart attack or myocardial infarction:* damage to some of the heart muscle due to lack of blood supply from blockage of a coronary artery or due to some severe stress such as malignant phase hypertension (not pulmonary hypertension). Heart attacks are not caused by scleroderma unless there is an episode of malignant phase hypertension (see Chapter 8, on scleroderma and the kidneys).

# 12
✳ ✳ ✳

# SCLERODERMA AND
# JOINTS, TENDONS,
# MUSCLES, AND NERVES

Stiffness and achiness are common problems in scleroderma. Sometimes patients can't tell whether the aching
is coming from the joints, the muscles, both, or neither.
The thickness and tightness of the overlying skin can make
it hard even for the doctor to determine if joint swelling is
present. This can be an important distinction to make, since
joint pain and swelling (arthritis) may require different treatment than muscle aches or tendon inflammation. A small
percentage of patients will have a true overlap between
rheumatoid arthritis and scleroderma and may need to be
treated with medications that are usually considered to be
specific for rheumatoid arthritis. Most, however, will not
have this overlap.

## *Joint Stiffness and Arthritis*

Many scleroderma patients have hand stiffness that is most marked in the morning, may or may not be associated with joint swelling, and improves with motion during the day. The swelling is not confined to the joints or knuckles of the hands but involves the whole fingers and sometimes the back of the hands as well. The entire hand seems "puffy." The patient cannot make a tight fist, a result of the excess fluid that also causes the puffiness. Many women compare it to fluid retention that commonly occurs just before the menstrual period. This is known as the *edematous phase* of scleroderma. It is not arthritis; the puffiness is due to damage to small blood vessels that make them leaky, so that excess fluid accumulates in the fingers and hands. This is seldom improved with diuretics, or "water pills," since the underlying problem is not fluid imbalance but damaged blood vessels. This edematous phase can last anywhere from weeks to years but does tend to improve on its own. Frequently it is replaced by a more lasting phase characterized by thickened and tightened skin that causes the fingers to curl down.

True joint stiffness is caused by inflammation in the joints. This can happen in scleroderma patients and is characterized by stiffness in many joints, including the hands, wrists, elbows, shoulders, knees, and ankles. There may or may not be noticeable swelling. The stiffness is worse on waking up and is improved by activity but can recur during the day after periods of inactivity such as riding in a car or sitting in a doctor's waiting room. In order to diagnose the problem, I often ask people if they are stiff when they first get up, and, if so, how long this morning stiffness lasts. (The phenomenon of sitting down and stiffening up again doesn't count in this determination.)

Osteoarthritis (the most common form of arthritis, affecting almost everyone as they get older) is characterized by morning stiffness lasting less than 30 minutes and frequently less than ten minutes. Inflammatory arthritis (such as rheumatoid arthritis and the mildly inflammatory arthritis that accompanies scleroderma and lupus) is characterized by morning stiffness lasting longer than 30 minutes, sometimes several hours. Inflammatory arthritis can be treated with several different types of medication, including the nonsteroidal anti-inflammatory drugs (NSAIDs). One of the potential side effects of this type of medicine is stomach irritation, which can be a problem in individuals with scleroderma who are already prone to GI upset. Some of the newer arthritis medicines are easier on the stomach but can still cause GI problems. In addition, all these medicines should be avoided or used with caution if there is kidney damage.

## Joint Contractures

Each joint has a normal range of motion, that is, it can be flexed inward, extended outward, or rotated. The elbow, for example, can be extended out straight to 180 degrees and flexed or bent in to about 30 degrees. It can't go any farther because the muscle tissue of the forearm hits the muscle tissue of the upper arm. Contracture of a joint means that the joint cannot be fully flexed or extended; it has lost some of its range of motion. When this occurs due to several different processes, the joints usually develop flexion contractures, in which the joint will not extend fully.

In scleroderma, the fingers tend to be flexed inward toward the palm and the wrists tend to lose motion in both directions. The elbows may not straighten out fully, and the shoulders can lose motion, so the arms cannot be extended through the normal arc of motion. Maintaining motion may require exercises on a daily basis to keep as much mobility as possible. Although this occurs in many patients, it does not happen in all. This is an important point to keep in mind as you read this book.

### Tendonitis and Tendon Rubs

A tendon is a fibrous cord that attaches a muscle to a bone. Tendons are enclosed in a tendon sheath that contains a small amount of fluid to provide for smooth gliding motion. A bursa is a small fluid-filled sac that overlies bony prominences. Tendonitis and bursitis are common problems in the general population, as evidenced by the following nicknames for these conditions: tennis elbow (inflammation of a tendon at the bony protuberance known as the medial epicondyle of the elbow; the condition is also called medial epicondylitis), housemaid's knee (inflammation of the bursa, a padlike sac containing fluid, over the kneecap, also known as prepatellar bursitis), and weaver's bottom (inflammation of the bursa over the "sit-bones," also known as ischial bursitis). However, scleroderma patients get a form of tendonitis that is not usually seen in the general population. The term *tendon rub* describes a sound like two pieces of leather rubbing together; this occurs when a tendon moves in an inflamed, roughened tendon sheath. This happens most commonly at the elbows, the knees, and the ankles. The condition is annoying rather than crippling. The treatment may involve applying heat, taking an NSAID medication, low-dose prednisone pills, and occasional injection of steroids into the area.

## Muscles: Polymyositis and Myopathy

Some scleroderma patients have a persistently abnormal elevation of a muscle enzyme, creatine phosphokinase (CPK or CK), in the blood. This substance comes from the breakdown of muscle, and higher-than-normal levels in the blood imply that muscle is breaking down at a faster-than-normal rate. (Some muscle tissue always breaks down and new muscle is made as part of the body's dynamic equilibrium, so a low level of CPK in the blood is normal.)

There is another autoimmune connective tissue disease known as polymyositis or dermatomyositis (polymyositis accompanied by a particular type of skin rash), which can be seen as an overlap with scleroderma. Symptoms include muscle weakness in the shoulder area and thighs. Although many scleroderma patients will have a sense of overall weakness and fatigue, this condition is distinct. The weakness is usually painless, and people may ignore it at first. In polymyositis, the CPK level in the blood is extremely elevated, sometimes ten times normal. Another muscle enzyme, aldolase, may also be abnormally high. Without treatment, the muscle inflammation can progress to cause destruction of muscles; in very extreme cases it can affect the muscles needed for breathing. It is important to treat this form of polymyositis with medication, usually steroids (cortisonelike medication) alone or steroids plus other immunosuppressive drugs (such as methotrexate or azathioprine). A muscle biopsy may be needed to confirm the diagnosis. This condition tends to have periods of exacerbation and remission, requiring treatment for several months to control the disease, after which the treatment can be stopped for a period of time that may last for months or years.

The other muscle problem that can occur with scleroderma is nonprogressive scleroderma myopathy. The CPK level in the blood is only modestly elevated (in the range of two to three times normal), and there is little or no muscle weakness. This condition does not affect the respiratory muscles and does not need medication. A muscle biopsy may show that collagen has replaced some muscle fibers, but there is little or no inflammation.

### Nerves

Nerve or neurological involvement in scleroderma comes in several different forms. These include entrapment neuropathies, cranial neuropathies, and peripheral sensorimotor neuropathies.

### Entrapment Neuropathies

Entrapment neuropathies occur when there is pressure put on a nerve, causing either pain or a tingling kind of numbness in the area that is supplied by the nerve. The most common form of entrapment neuropathy in the general population and in scleroderma patients is carpal tunnel syndrome. One of the major nerves to the hands is called the median nerve and goes through a narrow tunnel (the carpal tunnel) at the base of the palm. If this area becomes narrowed, by swelling from wrist arthritis, tendonitis, or other causes, pain or numbness will occur. This happens a lot in pregnant women, who tend to have swelling in both hands and feet; fortunately, it usually resolves spontaneously after delivery. Diabetics are prone to get this, too, as are people with rheumatoid arthritis involving the wrists. Scleroderma patients get it due to the swelling from leaking blood vessels, mentioned above, or from scar tissue buildup. The symptoms are numbness and tingling in the thumb, index, and long fingers, which tends to be worse at night and can awaken people from sleep. Sometimes it is difficult to distinguish between the tingling from Raynaud's phenomenon and the tingling from carpal tunnel syndrome. The usual way to figure this out is that Raynaud's tingling happens in response to cold exposure, and carpal-tunnel-related tingling happens when there is no change in temperature.

Other nerves can get trapped as well. The ulnar nerve, the nerve that is responsible for the "funny bone" feeling when you hit your elbow and get a painful shock that travels down into the little finger, gets very close to the skin surface when it goes around the elbow. In scleroderma the skin can get very tight at the elbow, the tendons shorten, and the elbow cannot be straightened out all the way. Sometimes the tightness is so severe that it presses on the nerve and causes pain down the forearm and into the little finger.

What can be done about entrapment neuropathies? For carpal tunnel syndrome or median nerve compression, wrist splints are recommended to hold the wrist and hand in the best position to open up the narrowed tunnel. Cortisone injections are sometimes used to relieve the inflammation that the pressure causes. In severe circumstances, surgery can be performed to open up the tunnel. Surgery can be done for ulnar neuropathy (at the elbow), but it is less successful than the carpal tunnel surgery and so should be approached with caution.

### Cranial Neuropathies

The cranial nerves are those that go to the head and are responsible for moving the muscles of the face and eyes and for providing sensation to these areas. Problems with these nerves are more often seen in lupus but can also occur in scleroderma. Occasionally scleroderma can cause a condition called *Bell's palsy*, which results in a droop of the face on one side. Bell's palsy can be caused by many different conditions (sometimes a virus) and may respond to prednisone (also known as cortisone) treatment.

Scleroderma can be associated with a painful condition called *trigeminal neuralgia,* or *tic douloureux* (painful spasm). This is caused by inflammation of the nerve that is responsible for providing sensation to one side of the face. When this nerve becomes inflamed, it causes pain that can wax and wane in intensity, sometimes being sharp and sometimes causing a pins-and-needles or numb sensation. If this condition does not respond to medication like prednisone, does not resolve on its own, and is very severe, the nerve may need to be surgically cut. This leaves an area of the face permanently numb, but numbness may be preferable to persistent or recurrent pain.

## Peripheral Sensorimotor Neuropathies

Sometimes nerves in other areas of the body will be affected, leading to numbness or tingling in a pattern that is different from the carpal tunnel syndrome or ulnar nerve problems mentioned above in the section on entrapment neuropathies. Occasionally there will also be weakness of a muscle that can cause a foot drop, that is, the inability to pick up the toes when walking. This is usually due to vasculitis, which is an inflammation of a blood vessel. If there is so much inflammation in the blood vessel that supplies nutrition to a nerve, the nerve can weaken and die. The diagnosis is usually made based on the patient's symptoms, as well as with an electromyogram (EMG) and nerve conduction tests (NCT). Since the underlying problem is inflammation, the treatment is medication such as steroids (cortisone or prednisone) or other immunosuppressive medications that combat inflammation. The nonsteroidal anti-inflammatory medicines (NSAIDs) are usually not strong enough to be helpful in this situation.

## Fibrositis or Fibromyalgia

Some scleroderma patients are also bothered with fibrositis or fibromyalgia. These two terms refer to a painful condition characterized by tender areas, called trigger points, at the base of the neck, across the upper back and shoulders, the low back, the inside of the knees, and the inside of the elbows. Fibromyalgia is associated with poor sleep patterns and sometimes with depression or anxiety. It is not clear if the pain starts first and then interferes with sleep or if the abnormal sleep pattern comes first and causes the muscle tenderness, but what is clear is that the pain and poor sleep go hand in hand.

Fibromyalgia is a very common condition in the general population, affecting people of all age groups. The treatment is usually a combination of physical therapy along with medication to improve sleep patterns or to relieve depression.

### *Physical Therapy*

The role of physical therapy in the treatment of scleroderma varies from one person to the next. Most individuals benefit from a program that teaches them about range-of-motion exercises they can do in their own home. Muscles that do not move will weaken and shrink (atrophy). The difficult part (as with all exercise programs) is to maintain a schedule of regular exercise for the long term.

As mentioned above, wrist splints can help with symptoms of carpal tunnel syndrome, and hand splints, used at night, may be useful to prevent or slow down flexion contractures of the fingers. Inflammatory arthritis of the hand joints may be helped by heat treatments, such as hot wax baths, but these should not be used if finger sores are present.

An exercise program has more benefits than just increased strength, improved mobility, and longer endurance. Exercise improves mood, helps restore normal sleep patterns, and results in a better sense of well-being and independence.

Some people get discouraged because they can no longer perform at the level they maintained prior to their illness. Just because you cannot run marathons does not mean you cannot walk daily, ride an exercise bike, or participate in a pool exercise program. Yoga can be a wonderful way to exercise the body and help calm the mind. There are now yoga classes and videotapes that are modified for the physically challenged. My yoga instructor has given presentations at the local Scleroderma Foundation chapter meeting that were met with great enthusiasm. She clearly did not know what she was getting into when I signed up for her class.

# 13

**❋ ❋ ❋**

# SYSTEMIC SCLERODERMA
# AND PREGNANCY

Young women with systemic scleroderma often ask me if it is okay to get pregnant. The answer is that it depends on several factors: the stage of the disease, the medications that are required to control the disease, and the risks that people are willing to take in order to have a child. (Note that this does not apply to people with localized scleroderma, a condition that does not present a higher-than-usual risk during pregnancy. However, the use of any medication needs to be reviewed by the patient and her doctor before pregnancy occurs.)

Pregnancy is a strain on the body even for individuals who are otherwise well. Even a normal pregnancy in a healthy individual can be complicated by high blood pressure, diabetes, kidney problems, circulation problems, heartburn, hemorrhoids, and a host of other difficulties. Pregnancy in a scleroderma patient has particular problems and is considered a high-risk condition, requiring careful monitoring of the mother and the baby. Many of my patients have successfully gotten pregnant, had a medically uneventful course, and delivered healthy babies. Others have not been this fortunate. Pregnancy has different effects on people with different connective tissue diseases. For example, in most cases pregnancy makes rheumatoid arthritis better and lupus worse. There does not seem to be a consistent effect on scleroderma patients; some do quite well and others do not.

It is important to consider the risks before contemplating pregnancy. If a patient has been diagnosed recently, I suggest that she wait to get pregnant for at least two or three years, to get a better idea of what type of scleroderma she has. Limited scleroderma presents less risk than diffuse disease, although there is some increase in blood pressure and risk of kidney problems in both types. People with diffuse disease run a greater risk of blood pressure problems, kidney disease, and heart disease.

Problems for the baby that can occur in scleroderma pregnancies include stillbirth, miscarriages, and low birth weight. Problems for the mother include serious blood pressure problems with the risk of kidney failure, strokes, and heart problems. There is a condition called preeclampsia that can occur in the absence of scleroderma but is somewhat more common in scleroderma patients. This condition is characterized by severe high blood pressure, swelling of the legs, and kidney damage. If preeclampsia is left untreated, it can progress to eclampsia, which causes seizures and is associated with a high mortality for both mothers and babies. The main treatment for preeclampsia is to deliver the baby, even though premature. In scleroderma the source of the problem is damage to the blood vessels in the placenta, which is the sac that surrounds the baby, provides it with nutrition and oxygen, and removes wastes. In this disease these blood vessels become thickened and narrowed, much like blood vessels elsewhere in the body.

The decision whether to have a child is a serious one that should be made after gathering information and discussing it with your loved ones, as there are several issues involved.

### Getting Pregnant

Women with scleroderma, like all women with a chronic disease, may have a harder time getting pregnant than their healthier counterparts. Menstrual abnormalities or irregular periods may be a sign that ovulation (the production of eggs) may not be occurring in a normal fashion. It is generally true, not just for scleroderma patients, that the longer one waits to become pregnant, the more difficult it can be to conceive.

Very little is known about the risks of using fertility drugs in people who have scleroderma. Since 80 percent of scleroderma patients are female, and since it is thought that female (estrogen-type) hormones play some role in the susceptibility to scleroderma, fertility drugs may be dangerous in scleroderma patients since they induce a high-estrogen state.

Also, some medications used for scleroderma can contribute to infertility. Drugs such as prednisone (a form of cortisone) can cause menstrual irregularities and decreased fertility. Other medicines such as cyclophosphamide can contribute to the onset of early menopause. Certain medications may not affect a woman's ability to get pregnant but could cause damage to the fetus (the developing baby) if they were taken during pregnancy. This is why it is very important to consult with your doctor about your desire to have a baby before you actually get pregnant. Most medications would have to be stopped before it would be safe to conceive a child.

Because of this requirement to stop medications, it is important that the scleroderma be stable, with no evidence of high blood pressure or active pulmonary disease, before getting pregnant. Women with preexisting pulmonary hypertension (PAH) or heart muscle dysfunction should probably avoid pregnancy. Women with some forms of heart conduction defects (a blocked heart rhythm) may still safely get pregnant, as long as the heart rhythm can be controlled by a pacemaker. Medications to prevent reflux (heartburn) need to be stopped as well. This may mean worse heartburn, but antacids can be safely substituted. Each patient is different.

## The Course of Pregnancy

Pregnancy in a scleroderma patient should always be considered high risk and followed by an obstetrician familiar with such high-risk situations, in collaboration with the treating rheumatologist. Ideally medications will have been stopped before the pregnancy occurred. Certainly once a woman is pregnant, the usual scleroderma medications have to be stopped in order to prevent problems for the baby.

The normal nausea or morning sickness in early pregnancy can be exaggerated in some scleroderma patients. Individuals need to check their blood pressure frequently, twice a week or even daily, to make sure that it stays under good control. If the blood pressure goes up, medication needs to be given to lower it. There are some blood pressure medicines that are safer than others during pregnancy, and the usual type of medicine to lower scleroderma-related high blood pressure, an ACE inhibitor, is not given unless other medicines cannot adequately manage the situation.

If severe hypertension (preeclampsia) occurs and the blood pressure cannot be adequately controlled by medication, then the baby needs to be delivered, usually by cesarean section and regardless of the degree of prematurity. This is the most dangerous complication for scleroderma patients and for the baby. This is one of those "what if" situations that the patient, along with her family and her doctor, needs to address prior to or early in the course of the pregnancy. It can be a difficult and sad situation, but individuals need to weigh the risks and benefits and decide what is best for them.

Heartburn is a common and almost universal symptom in pregnancy, even for those without scleroderma, so it is easy to understand that it will be especially pronounced in those with the disease. The proton pump inhibitors are not usually given in pregnancy, making this problem extra difficult. Antireflux measures such as elevating the head of the bed, avoiding eating in the two hours before bedtime, avoiding caffeine, and using antacids are helpful.

Is there any good news in all of this? Well, actually there is. Raynaud's phenomenon usually improves in pregnancy. A small point, perhaps, but most people enjoy this.

*Labor and Delivery*

For the most part, once the pregnancy has reached term, labor and delivery are no different for the scleroderma patient than for anyone else.

## Case Histories

One of my patients, now in her midtwenties, has had systemic scleroderma from the age of 11. She was quite sick in the first few years and had malignant phase hypertension and kidney problems, all of which were treated promptly. She recovered 90 percent of her kidney function. Her skin has returned almost totally to normal in terms of skin thickness and tightness, but she has quite a few telangiectasias (red spots) on her face, arms, legs, and trunk. She still has some reflux symptoms and has Raynaud's attacks. Her blood pressure "acts up" about twice a year, requiring treatment with an ACE inhibitor for a few months. She has no evidence of heart or lung involvement. She wanted to get pregnant, so I advised her to stop her medication first and see how things went for a few months. All was well, so she went ahead and got pregnant.

Just a few weeks ago she was in my office to show off the baby, now ten months old. She had problems during her pregnancy with blood pressure, which was treated successfully with no damage to her kidneys. She had a cesarean section (probably unrelated to the scleroderma) at the end of a full-term pregnancy and is doing just fine.

Not everyone is so lucky. Another patient, in her early thirties, had systemic scleroderma for six years. By all measures the disease was stable, with no development of new heart, lung, blood pressure, or kidney problems for about two years. She and her husband were both eager to have children. Late in the second trimester, at about six months, she developed malignant phase hypertension that could not be controlled, and she went into kidney failure and lost the baby. She is now on dialysis, some four years later, and is considering a kidney transplant. She and her husband have since adopted a child.

Another of my patients, with both diffuse scleroderma and rheumatoid arthritis, decided to adopt rather than run the risk of a pregnancy.

Many scleroderma patients successfully get pregnant, have healthy babies, and do very well. Other individuals decide to forgo pregnancy because of the risk of damaging their own health and losing the baby. Every case is different, and it is an individual decision. Parenthood is one of the greatest joys in life and also one of the greatest responsibilities. Although the facts presented in this chapter may be sobering, there is no right decision for all. Any decision, however, should be an informed one.

# 14

**\* \* \***

# SCLERODERMA
# AND SEXUALITY

Sexuality involves the physiological and the psychological, the body and the mind. These two features are always intertwined in human behavior, but this is particularly true in the realm of sexuality. This chapter is divided into three sections: on women, on men, and on partners.

### Women, Scleroderma,
### and Sexuality

Physical problems for women with scleroderma include fatigue, dryness of the vagina (as part of Sjogren's syndrome), and physical discomfort during sex that is a result of decreased mobility of joints, sometimes associated with joint pain. Also, symptoms of reflux (heartburn) can be worsened by lying flat and by having the weight of a body on top. Depression, which usually causes lack of libido or desire, can add to this problem.

## *Fatigue*

Fatigue is a common problem in the general population. Sometimes it is difficult to distinguish the fatigue that is associated with depression or hopelessness from the fatigue that commonly accompanies a connective tissue disease. My patients frequently tell me that it is all they can do to go to work each day or to get household chores done, much less have extra energy to devote to their families in the evening. What frequently goes unstated is that this level of fatigue also means there is not enough energy to enjoy an active sexual relationship with their partner. Women seldom bring this up. Fatigue is considered a personal problem, a fault, a failing. Fatigued people are thought of as "lazy" or simply as lacking the motivation to get things done.

Also, fatigue tends to develop gradually and is sometimes unnoticed until either medication is given or the disease begins to stabilize. Patients will then comment to me that they are feeling better and suddenly have their energy back again.

From a doctor's point of view, fatigue is a difficult symptom to treat. There is no medication that will magically make it go away and restore energy. My advice is to stop beating yourself up over it. I have a patient who tells me that she has a Plan A and a Plan B. Plan A is for the days when her energy level is good. In addition to her necessary activities, she can take on some extra projects. Plan B is for the days when she knows she has to take it easy. She considers Plan B days as those for rest and restoration. She has had more Plan A days than Plan B days over the course of her illness, but she tries to avoid labeling them as "good days" and "bad days." Both are part of the ebb and flow of her life now. She is fortunate in having an understanding family who are keyed into the plans. If there is a special outing scheduled, she rests up to prepare herself for it. This outlook on life requires the confidence that there will be Plan A days and the acceptance that Plan B days happen and are okay.

I wish I could take this attitude and transplant it into others. But too often it happens that constant fatigue can nudge people into depression. Fatigue and depression are closely interrelated—fatigue can lead to depression, just as depression is usually associated with fatigue. A patient whom I saw recently was complaining bitterly about her fatigue. She has five-year-old twins, as well as two school-age children. She had to quit her job due to her fatigue. Even without working outside the home, she was still tired a great deal. I tried to point out to her that just being home with her children was a gift to them, but she didn't buy it. She complained that her older children sometimes had to help her out with the younger ones. I said it would teach them responsibility, but she was stuck. All she could see was her shortcomings. She was unable to get pleasure from what she was able to do.

This is a common feature of depression. Depressed individuals are unable to see the whole picture. They are blocked from enjoyment, and no amount of persuasion will convince them otherwise. Persistent depression like this may require professional help as well as medication.

If sex is important to your relationship (as it usually is), then resting up for it or planning for it may become necessary. Although this may take away some of the spontaneity, the rewards of having an active sex life will make up for this. For many couples, especially those in long-term relationships, the need for cuddling, hugs, and general physical contact short of intercourse, is an essential part of their connection. Not all expressions of affection lead to sex and it is important to maintain this sense of closeness.

## Vaginal Dryness

Sjogren's syndrome frequently accompanies systemic scleroderma. This causes dryness of the mucous membranes, typically leading to symptoms of dry eyes and dry mouth. The vagina can also become dry, with less lubrication during arousal, making sex uncomfortable or even painful. Vaginal lubricants that can be purchased in most drugstores are very helpful. However, before you blame scleroderma and Sjogren's syndrome, it is important to realize that vaginal dryness can also occur with menopause and the drop of female hormones that accompanies it. If this is the case, either estrogen replacement hormones in pill form or an estrogen-containing vaginal cream can be useful.

## Estrogen Hormone Use
## and Scleroderma

I am often asked by scleroderma patients about the safety of estrogen, either in birth control pills or as hormone replacement after menopause. After all, since most scleroderma patients are women, doesn't it make sense to avoid these medicines? The answer to this question is not that simple and the decision needs to be individualized for each patient.

In terms of birth control pills, there is no good evidence that these are harmful in scleroderma. Individuals who have a family history of breast or uterine cancer, or who have a problem with blood clotting should avoid estrogen use. However, these precautions apply to all women; not just to scleroderma patients.

The issue of estrogens as hormone replacement therapy after menopause is a difficult one. Again, there is no good evidence that this makes scleroderma worse. However, there are other reasons to be cautious about taking this. For women who still have their uterus (women who have not had a hysterectomy), hormone replacement must be a combination of estrogen and progesterone. There is now fairly good evidence that this hormone combination can increase the risk of breast cancer over time. On the good side, this form of treatment does help prevent osteoporosis, the loss of bone that can lead to fractures as women get older. There are other approaches to prevent osteoporosis including calcium, exercise, and nonestrogen medicines. Do the risks outweigh the benefits? You need to talk this over with your doctor and make a decision that is right for you individually.

Is the use of estrogens safe in women who have had a hysterectomy and who can take estrogen alone, without the addition of progesterone? Currently this seems to be the case, and studies are in progress to better answer this question. Again, estrogen does not seem to worsen (or improve) scleroderma, so the decision to start this medicine or to continue taking it should be made on an individual basis.

## Joint Discomfort

Some women find sex painful because they have trouble finding a comfortable position. Joints are stiff and sore, or limbs just don't move the way they used to. A warm bath may help to loosen up joints. The real resolution to this problem is imagination, creativity, a sense of humor, and a loving partner.

## Emotional and Psychological Issues

Emotional and psychological issues also get in the way of sexual enjoyment. These include depression, which typically decreases sex drive; changes in body image, leading to the fear that you are not as attractive as before; and anxiety that sex will be painful. Male partners of women with scleroderma can be affected by this attitude of heightened anxiety and retreat from sex for fear of causing pain and discomfort in the women they love. In the absence of good communication, both partners can fall into a world of silence that fosters isolation and loneliness. This is an area where a counselor can be tremendously helpful. If one of the partners is reluctant to talk about such personal issues in the presence of a "stranger," the other partner can go alone and talk about fears of the illness and what it means for both partners and their future. The real issue is communication, more so than the technical aspects of sexual intercourse. Once communication is reestablished, the rest can follow.

Depression has been called "anger turned inward." There are many reasons to be angry at the disease, at the limitations it places on your life, at the unfairness in getting it, at the burden you feel it places on your family. When the anger is turned inward on yourself, you can get feelings of worthlessness and defeat. When the anger is turned outward toward those closest to you (which is typically the case since they are handy), you can drive away the very people who love you most.

The first step in dealing with any of these issues is to acknowledge that they exist, that your feelings are valid and understandable, and that the disease *is not your fault*. Each person reacts to this new reality in different ways, but I have yet to meet someone who can accept the diagnosis and go away unchanged. The challenge is to manage the change in a way that makes you more connected to yourself and to those who love you.

### Men, Scleroderma, and Sexuality

I have stated several times in this book that 80 percent of scleroderma patients are women. This, obviously, leaves 20 percent that are men. I have seen and treated over 1,000 scleroderma patients, which means that I have seen approximately 200 male patients. The most common complaint I hear from male patients regarding sexual problems involves impotence, particularly the ability to get and maintain an erection. This is not the only concern, of course. It is not surprising that men are also worried about body image, about being attractive to their partners, about their ability to keep a job and provide for their families. Fatigue and depression are significant problems. But erectile dysfunction (ED) is seen as insult heaped on injury. It is not unfair enough for them to get a "woman's disease" but it also strikes at a key function of maleness that seems particularly unjust. There are several physiological explanations for the ED that can accompany scleroderma. These include neurological abnormalities, vascular problems, medication side effects, and psychological and emotional difficulties.

## Neurological Abnormalities

The penis becomes erect when more blood is directed into it than is drained from it. This requires the coordinated action of blood vessels and nerves. The part of the nervous system that is responsible for this is called the sympathetic nervous system, which is part of a network that transmits signals from the brain to various parts of the body. There is some evidence from medical research that the sympathetic nervous system can be damaged in scleroderma, and this may account for difficulties with erection in some patients.

## Vascular Problems

Vascular problems are common in scleroderma. Damage to blood vessels is what causes Raynaud's phenomenon, finger sores, and high blood pressure. The blood supply to the penis can also be affected.

The key issue is what can be done about it. Unfortunately, once the damage is done to the blood vessels or to the nerves, it may not be possible to reverse it. As anyone who lives in the United States and has a television knows, there are now two approved medications (sildenafil or Viagra, and tadalafil or Cialis) that increase circulation to the penis and improve erectile function. I recommend that patients discuss the alternatives with their doctor, who may suggest a consultation with a urologist who is also a specialist in problems of erectile disfunction. Besides medication, there are external devices that can be applied to the penis to stimulate an erection; these may work for some people. There are also implantable devices that can be used. The point is that there are treatments for this problem. An added benefit is that these medications may improve Raynaud's attacks as well, although they are not approved for this indication.

## Medication Side Effects

Problems with erections can also be the result of side effects from medication. This is occasionally seen with a common medication that is used to treat Raynaud's phenomenon and finger ulcers, namely, nifedipine or other calcium channel blockers. It is paradoxical that medications used to improve the circulation to the fingers can result in impaired circulation to the penis, but this is sometimes the case. I would strongly suggest that you discuss the issue with your doctor before stopping the medication and that you get a workup by a urologist.

## Psychological and Emotional Difficulties

Psychological and emotional problems also play a key role in sexual function. A decrease in sex drive (libido) commonly occurs with fatigue and depression. Fatigue can be a feature of all connective tissue diseases (rheumatoid arthritis, lupus, and scleroderma). As noted above, some people dismiss the fatigue as "laziness" and think that if they just push themselves harder, it will go away. But listen to your body. If it is telling you that you need more rest, then you need more rest.

Depression can also deprive people of the ability to enjoy life, and along with this may come loss of libido. There are many reasons for depression, and none should be dismissed out of hand. Many of my male patients have expressed concern over holding their jobs, and they frequently will not tell their employers of their illness if this is at all possible. Accepting disability or a decreased level of activity is difficult emotionally for many men, especially if it is associated with a loss of income. Some men feel guilty for bringing economic hardship to their families. Wives may resent bearing the burden of supporting the family. Although these feelings are not unique to men (many of my women patients express the same concerns), it is still true that men, more so than women, tend to define themselves by the job they do and their sense of self-worth is strongly associated with work performance.

There is another feature of scleroderma that is unique for men. Most of my male patients have told me at one time or another that they resent having a "female" disease. In this culture, men are not supposed to get sick; if sick, they are not supposed to dwell on it. Given this, it may be exceptionally difficult for a man to disclose that he has scleroderma and then hear the response "Oh, I thought that was a woman's disease." But the fact that scleroderma affects mostly women does not mean that a man who has it is less than male. Male hormone levels are normal in scleroderma patients; sperm production is good, and male patients can father children. In other words, there is no apparent defect in "maleness" caused by or related to scleroderma.

One additional problem that can occur with male scleroderma patients is that a band of thickened skin can develop on the side of the penis and interfere with erection and/or make the erect penis crooked. If mild, nothing needs to be done. If severe enough to interfere with intercourse, then a surgical procedure can be done to remove some of this scar tissue and straighten the penis.

### Spouses, Scleroderma, and Sexuality

So your spouse has scleroderma. What does this mean for you? It means that life is different from what it used to be. All things of importance that happen to you affect your relationship with your spouse, and the same is true of important things that happen to her or him. Certainly if you changed jobs, decided to become a vegetarian, or converted to a different religion, it would have an impact on your spouse. All of these things profoundly affect your day-to-day activities, your view of the world, and your view of yourself. Getting a rare, incurable, and chronic disease is one of those life-changing events. The difference between this and other life changes is that getting this disease is nonvoluntary. You can hope that your spouse will have a mild form of scleroderma, with little impact on usual activities and no impact on longevity, but you can't count on it.

You can call it unfair, and you will be right. You can protest that your life should not have to change, and you will be wrong. If you are too busy, then you will have to let something else go. If you can't handle it alone, then you must get help. You may feel that your spouse is too demanding, is wallowing in self-pity, or is exaggerating symptoms. This may actually be the case. If so, then both of you need to work out your feelings of disappointment, resentment, anger at the disease, or whatever is behind this behavior.

Sometimes the unaffected partner can develop an "Oh, you poor thing! Let me do that for you" attitude toward his or her spouse. But pity takes away responsibility, robs individuals of the means to influence their own lives, and turns them into passive recipients dependent on the goodwill of others. Pity may feel good in the short term, but it is poison in the long term. Just because someone needs help in some areas of living does not mean that they are helpless. Resentment in this situation frequently goes both ways.

Striking a new balance in a relationship is a very difficult thing to do. People get used to their roles and resent change, especially change that is forced upon them by circumstances beyond their control. But change can also be a challenge, an opportunity, a chance to reexamine what is important in life.

I have seen marriages become stronger in the face of this type of adversity. Unfortunately, I have also watched marriages fall apart. In the latter case, it is usually because the relationship was rocky before the onset of illness—communication was poor to begin with, and one or both partners were not committed to making things work. The illness then becomes the excuse for the breakup, but the real reasons go much deeper. Whatever your personal situation, know that you cannot successfully address these issues alone. Turn to your loved ones for support. Get professional help if you need it. If you cannot afford it or if your insurance does not cover this type of service, you can turn to your church or synagogue. Most priests, ministers, or rabbis can offer support or can suggest where such support can be found.

# 15

**❋ ❋ ❋**

# OVERLAP SYNDROMES
# AND
# SCLERODERMALIKE
# CONDITIONS

I n most cases, the autoimmune connective tissue diseases—
rheumatoid arthritis, lupus, scleroderma, polymyositis,
and dermatomyositis—occur as separate entities. Occasionally, more than one of these diseases will coexist in the same
patient, and these people are said to have overlap syndromes,
with features of two or more diseases. Sjogren's syndrome (dry
eyes and dry mouth) is the exception in that it usually coex-
ists with the above diseases, although there are cases when it
occurs alone. Sometimes one connective tissue disease will
exist by itself for several years before the features of another
condition develop. This tends to cause confusion in people
who, having been told that they have one disease, are then
told that they have another. Since many symptoms are similar among these diseases, making the diagnosis of one versus another can be difficult, particularly in the early stages.

## Mixed Connective Tissue Disease

Mixed connective tissue disease, or MCTD, is a combination of lupus, scleroderma, and polymyositis along with a positive blood test for an antibody to ribonucleic protein (RNP). RNP is a protein that is attached to RNA, or ribonucleic acid, part of the machinery in the cell for manufacturing proteins from the genetic code of DNA. It is not clear why an antibody is produced to this protein, and it is not clear that this antibody actually plays any role in the development of the disease. There is only the observation that this antibody is seen in association with MCTD and serves as a useful test to help make the diagnosis.

In order to explain this condition, it may be helpful to describe a patient. I first saw one young woman about ten years ago. She had diffuse scleroderma with a lot of skin involvement. At that time her ANA (antinuclear antibody) was positive, as it is in 85 to 90 percent of scleroderma patients and in 95 percent of lupus patients. However, she had no features of lupus. Her RNP antibody test was negative. About two years later she developed very severe muscle inflammation (polymyositis) and became so weak she had trouble walking. This inflammation improved with steroids (prednisone) and an immunosuppressive medication, and over the following two years she regained her strength but had problems with lung fibrosis. Two years later she developed fluid around her heart (pericarditis) and was admitted to the hospital to get the fluid drained. She also had vasculitis (inflammation of blood vessels) that produced a wrist drop that was more typical of lupus than of scleroderma. On repeat testing, she was shown to have RNP antibodies. In this case, her disease had started as classical scleroderma, and only later developed into polymyositis and then lupus.

MCTD can start as scleroderma, as lupus, or as polymyositis. It is unusual for features of all three diseases to be present at the beginning. The sequence of events will vary from one person to the next. Some people start out as lupus or as polymyositis, get treated for this condition, and may improve for a time, only to later develop signs of scleroderma. Because my practice is involved with treating scleroderma, I tend to see patients who start out as scleroderma and then develop the overlap.

### Scleroderma and Polymyositis

This is an overlap that occurs in about 25 percent of scleroderma patients. The polymyositis occurs as a gradual, and usually painless, muscle weakness that affects the shoulder muscles and the hip muscles more than the muscles of the hands or feet. The blood levels of muscle enzymes (CPK and aldolase) are increased, and a test of muscle function called an EMG will show evidence of muscle inflammation. A muscle biopsy may be needed to confirm the diagnosis. An MRI can be helpful to visualize the muscle inflammation to help make the diagnosis as well as to follow the course of the disease. Treatment usually consists of steroids and immunosuppressive agents. Frequently this treatment is needed for only one to two years and then can be gradually tapered and stopped without recurrence of muscle inflammation. In some cases, low doses of these medications are needed on a longer term basis to control the muscle disease.

Some scleroderma patients will have a modest elevation in muscle enzymes (CPK or aldolase) that does not
cause weakness, is not inflammatory, does not worsen over
time, and does not respond to treatment. This is called a
*myopathy* and does not need to be treated. Thyroid problems can also cause muscle weakness and an increase in
the blood levels of muscle enzymes. A simple blood test
(TSH or thyroid stimulating hormone) is frequently done
to check for this.

### Scleroderma and Rheumatoid Arthritis

These two diseases coexist in only 5 to 10 percent of scleroderma cases. It is not enough for the blood test for rheumatoid factor to be positive or for the joints to "ache." A
diagnosis of rheumatoid arthritis requires swelling of the
joint capsule and X-ray evidence of damage or erosions in
the joints. The treatment is the same as for rheumatoid arthritis without scleroderma and may include methotrexate, etanercept (Enbrel) inflixamab (Remicade), or
adalimumab (Humira).

### Scleroderma and Lupus

This is another unusual combination, occurring in about 5
percent of scleroderma cases. I did not think this condition
really existed until one of my patients proved me wrong.
She is an individual with limited scleroderma that began
almost 20 years ago. I have been following her for the last
eight years or so. She is doing quite well and continues to

work, and I had pretty much stopped worrying about her, seeing her every six months or so. She called one day and told me that her feet were swelling and that she just wasn't feeling very well. I saw her in the office and ordered some tests. To my surprise, she had protein and red cells in her urine and a positive anti-DNA antibody test (a test very specific for lupus). The protein loss in the urine was responsible for her swelling. A kidney biopsy confirmed lupus kidney disease, and she was treated for one year with steroids and immunosuppressives. The protein in her urine cleared up, her kidney function remains normal, and I am back to seeing her every six months.

This case also demonstrates a key difference between scleroderma and lupus. Lupus tends to have disease flares followed by remissions (usually due to treatment) lasting for months or years, followed by more flares. Scleroderma, on the other hand, tends to have a more chronic course.

### Scleroderma and Sjogren's Syndrome

This is a common combination. Sjogren's syndrome is characterized by dry mucous membranes, that is dry eyes, dry mouth, and in women a dry vagina. It is caused by an immune attack on the glands that produce mucus and saliva in these organs. Again, it is not known why the immune system becomes activated to recognize this target as foreign.

The lack of tears causes the eyes to feel dry, irritated, and "gritty." There can be dried secretions in the inner corner of the eye on awakening in the morning. If severe, there can be abrasions or ulcers that develop on the cornea, the clear covering over the pupil and iris, and this can eventually interfere with vision.

Lack of saliva causes the mouth to feel dry. However, there are many reasons for a dry mouth other than Sjogren's syndrome. Perhaps the most common cause of mouth dryness is the habit of breathing through the mouth, which occurs in people with allergies or sinus problems. Many medications, including over-the-counter ones, have dry mouth as a side effect. These include antihistamines, decongestants, some blood pressure pills, antidepressant medicines, and numerous others. The problem of decreased production of saliva is not just discomfort. Saliva helps to control the normal bacteria in the mouth and prevents tooth cavities. People with Sjogren's syndrome need to see a dentist more frequently and need to be more careful with brushing and flossing. This can be a difficult problem if the mouth cannot be opened wide due to scleroderma.

Lack of vaginal moisture and lubrication can make sexual intercourse uncomfortable and even painful. This is not always due to Sjogren's but can also occur after menopause, with the loss of estrogen. In some people it may be a combination of both conditions. Estrogen replacement, either by pills, skin patches, or a vaginal cream, can help if the dryness is primarily due to estrogen deficiency. The estrogen-containing vaginal creams appear to be safe and effective, however the pills and patches may not be.

The issue of estrogen replacement therapy in scleroderma patients after menopause is a difficult one. Although there is no good evidence that it makes scleroderma worse, there are other reasons to be cautious about taking the estrogen/progesterone combination. For women who still have their uterus (women who have not had a hysterectomy), hormone replacement must be a combination of estrogen and progesterone. There is now fairly good evidence that this hormone combination can increase the risk of breast cancer over time. On the good side, this form of treatment does help prevent osteoporosis, the loss of bone that can lead to fractures as women get older. There are other approaches to prevent osteoporosis including calcium, exercise, and nonestrogen medicines. Do the risks outweigh the benefits? You need to talk this over with your doctor and make a decision that is right for you individually.

Is the use of estrogens safe in women who have had a hysterectomy and who can take estrogen alone, without the addition of progesterone? Currently this seems to be the case, and studies are in progress to better answer this question. Again, estrogen does not seem to worsen (or improve) scleroderma, so the decision to start this medicine or to continue taking it should be made on an individual basis.

There are many over-the-counter preparations specifically formulated as vaginal lubricants that are very helpful. Petroleum jelly (Vaseline) and similar preparations are not recommended.

### Scleroderma and Thyroid Disease: Hashimoto's and Graves' Disease

Thyroid problems can result in an underactive thyroid (Hashimoto's thyroiditis) or an overactive thyroid (Graves' disease). Both of these conditions are caused by an immune attack on the thyroid tissue.

The thyroid gland is located in the front of the neck just below the Adam's apple. It controls the metabolic rate of the entire body. Typical symptoms of an underactive thyroid are weight gain, fatigue, dry skin, and constipation. Symptoms of an overactive thyroid are weight loss, diarrhea, jitteriness, and a fast heart rate. These symptoms can also be seen in scleroderma itself, and often occur in people without thyroid problems. Fortunately, there is a simple blood test that measures thyroid activity. An underactive thyroid condition is treated with thyroid replacement, while an overactive thyroid can be treated with medication to either control the symptoms or to prevent the gland from producing too much hormone.

### Scleroderma and Other Diseases

Just because you have scleroderma does not mean that you cannot get other conditions. The above overlap syndromes are particular situations. However, scleroderma patients can still get other common conditions such as colds, flu, bladder infections, and so on. In addition, people with scleroderma still have the same risk as those without scleroderma of developing more serious conditions such as breast cancer or uterine cancer. You still need routine checkups including Pap smears and breast exams for women, and prostate checks for men.

### Undifferentiated Connective Tissue Disease (UCTD)

Some people experience a few signs and symptoms, and even have some laboratory test abnormalities, that suggest they have a connective tissue disease, but the picture is incomplete. They "almost" have lupus or scleroderma, but not quite. They do not fit nicely into the diagnostic categories that the textbooks describe. It is wrong to diagnose such people as having scleroderma or lupus if they do not have these diseases. Rather, they are said to have undifferentiated connective tissue disease, or UCTD. In one study that followed a number of patients for many years, about one-third of people with UCTD went on to develop a defined disease (that is, they fulfilled the textbook definition), about one-third got better, and about one-third stayed in the "gray zone."

Although this may be an unsatisfactory diagnosis for some people, it is about as good as we can get in terms of accurately defining these diseases. In the future, when we find out what actually causes autoimmune diseases, we will be able to specify particular tests and provide a better diagnosis. Until then, UCTD will remain a possible diagnosis.


### Sclerodermalike Disorders

There are some conditions that resemble scleroderma but have certain features that are quite distinct. Because of these differences, they are usually classified as sclerodermalike disorders. These include eosinophilic fasciitis, sclerodema or scleromyxedema, chronic graft versus host disease, and eosinophilia myalgia syndrome.


#### Eosinophilic Fasciitis (EF)

In eosinophilic fasciitis (EF), white blood cells (*eosinophils* and *leukocytes*) attack the fascia, which is a thin sheet of tissue that separates muscle from the fat and skin above it. In some cases the fascia becomes inflamed, that is, it becomes swollen and tender. The skin overlying the fascia appears puckered, like the skin of an orange, and the tissue under the skin feels hard (some say that it feels like wood). Eosinophilic fasciitis affects the arms, legs, and trunk while sparing the hands and face, since there is little fascia in the hands and face. Also, contractures of the elbows or knees and decreased range of motion at the shoulders, hips, and central body occur rapidly, sometimes within a few weeks of the onset of the skin changes. This is more rapid than with scleroderma. Joint pains and carpal tunnel syndrome are frequently seen, which is also true in systemic scleroderma. Usually (but not always) there is no Raynaud's phenomenon, and the ANA is negative.

The diagnosis of EF is made on the basis of the pattern of skin involvement (for example, if the hands are affected early, it usually is not EF); on the basis of the appearance of the skin and feel of the tissue; and on a deep biopsy of skin, fat, and fascia. Sometimes a blood test will also show high levels of eosinophils, especially in the early stages of the condition.

The cause of this condition is not known. Eosinophils are a type of white blood cell that are important in allergic reactions and in some autoimmune diseases. A higher-than-normal eosinophil count is seen in some people with scleroderma, both systemic and localized. This does not mean that they are "allergic" to something; at least, we don't know what they are allergic to. Eosinophilic fasciitis is sometimes seen after a period of unusually heavy exercise or after significant trauma. In many cases, however, there is no apparent initiating event. Treatment consists of cortisone and immunosuppressive medications.

### Sclerodema or Scleromyxedema

Sclerodema, also known as scleromyxedema, is a condition characterized by thickened skin of the face, head, neck, and shoulders, sometimes extending down into the arms. It can also affect the trunk as well, although it usually spares the hands. Typically (but not always) there is no Raynaud's phenomenon, and the ANA is negative.

This condition is usually associated with long-standing diabetes or with a bone marrow abnormality that can be either benign (a monoclonal gammopathy that is not cancerous) or malignant (multiple myeloma that is cancerous). If the cause is diabetes, then it is important to get very tight control of the blood sugar. If the cause is a bone marrow abnormality, then treatment of the underlying disease will often improve the symptoms.

### Chronic Graft versus Host Disease (GVHD)

Graft versus host disease occurs in a very specific and unusual setting. It happens in some people who get bone marrow transplants as part of treatment for cancer. High-dose chemotherapy is first given to the patient to get rid of the cancer cells. The chemotherapy also results in the destruction of the patient's bone marrow, which is responsible for making red cells, white cells, and platelets. Since the white cells are killed off, the patient's immune system is also destroyed.

Following the chemotherapy, bone marrow taken from a matched donor is given to reconstitute the patient's (the host's) blood cells and immune system. The bone marrow has to be well matched so that the donor immune system cells will not recognize the host body tissue as foreign and mount an immune attack on it. In spite of an apparent match, sometimes there is an immediate and severe rejection reaction called acute graft versus host disease. This is treated with medication that suppresses the immune system and stops the rejection process.

In some cases there is a less severe form of rejection reaction that occurs over a period of months to years and consists of patches of thickened skin over the arms, legs, and trunk that is very similar to localized scleroderma. It is treated with some of the same medications that are used in acute graft versus host disease. The reaction can be controlled, but is seldom totally cured and therefore is termed chronic GVHD.

It should be noted that this reaction does not occur with kidney transplants, or other organ transplants since these organs do not contain immune cells. In the case of organ transplants the recipient's immune system is intact.

### *Eosinophilia Myalgia Syndrome (EMS)*

Eosinophilia myalgia syndrome (EMS) was first described in 1989 and occurred in a group of patients who had taken a health-food supplement with tryptophan that contained a contaminant, the nature of which is still uncertain. The health-food supplement was taken off the market, and the "epidemic" subsided. However, there are still occasional cases that occur in people who have never taken any tryptophan supplements. The condition is characterized by thickened and tight skin over the extremities (usually sparing the hands and feet), swelling of the extremities, rash, and pain in muscles and joints. Muscle pain is a very prominent feature of this condition. Additionally, nerves can be affected, causing burning and stinging sensations in multiple areas of the body. Lung problems occur in about half of affected people. Treatment for this condition consists of prednisone and immunosuppressive drugs, but the response is incomplete.

# IV

## COPING WITH SCLERODERMA

# 16

**✳ ✳ ✳**

# YOU AND
# YOUR DOCTOR

**P**rior to getting scleroderma, most patients have little knowledge about the medical profession and all its sub-specialties.

In the early period, soon after getting diagnosed, scleroderma patients are frequently uncertain about what kind of doctor they should see, so they rely on the advice of their general medical doctor. Most patients will benefit from an evaluation by a specialist who knows scleroderma, and most of the time this will be a rheumatologist. Whether or not the rheumatologist provides ongoing care after this evaluation will vary from case to case.

The initial workup usually includes the following:

*A comprehensive history and physical.* The history includes information on your past medical problems, on your Raynaud's attacks, on difficulties (or lack of difficulties) with heartburn or trouble breathing, and a long list of other questions. The physical part is pretty basic, with a close examination of your skin, particularly your fingertips; listening to your lungs and heart with the stethoscope; evaluation of joint mobility, and so on. No part of this phase of the workup involves anything especially fancy, painful, complicated, or expensive.

*Blood and urine tests.* This will vary depending on what your primary doctor has done and on what the rheumatologist finds on the history and physical, but may include routine tests of blood counts, kidney, liver, and muscle function, as well as a test for the autoantibodies (antinuclear antibodies, or ANA) typically seen in the connective tissue diseases.

*Baseline tests of internal organ involvement.* It is impossible to give a list of tests that would apply to every scleroderma patient. Potentially this could include tests to evaluate the function of the lungs, heart, esophagus, stomach, and bowel. Which tests are done depend on what symptoms people have. In most circumstances I like to get baseline tests of lung and heart function. Pulmonary function tests measure lung volumes, airflow, and air exchange from the lungs into the blood. They can pick up early scleroderma lung disease, even before there are any changes on the chest X-ray. An echocardiogram is an ultrasound test of the heart that shows how well both sides of the heart are pumping.

*Specialized tests of internal organ involvement.* If it is clear to me from the history and physical and/or from the baseline tests mentioned above that there is internal organ damage, the question then becomes how severe the damage is and whether it is progressive. In this case, special tests such as a high-resolution CAT scan of the lungs, cardiac catheterization, or others may be necessary. This may require referral to other subspecialists.

### Test after Test, Doctor after Doctor

My patients frequently express their frustration about having all these tests, each ordered, performed, and interpreted by a different doctor. They are confused as to the meaning of the results, and they worry that there is poor communication among their many physicians. Each doctor is prescribing something for one part of the body and seems to be uninterested in or, worse, less than knowledgeable about the process of scleroderma as a whole.

I wish I could offer an easy solution to this problem. The fact is that modern medicine is so complex that it is no longer possible for one physician to perform and interpret all the different tests (cardiac catheterization, stress tests, endoscopy, bronchoscopy, and others) and to know all the latest treatments for all the systems of the body. This is both good news and bad news. The good news is that today we can diagnose and treat hundreds of different conditions that could not be diagnosed accurately or treated effectively even a decade ago. The bad news is that you have to go to multiple doctors, undergo multiple tests (some "uncomfortable," which is the medical lingo for "painful"), and be confused by multiple and sometimes seemingly contradictory descriptions of what is wrong.

It is at this point that multiple doctors come into the picture and you, the patient, have to become actively involved in your care. The key issue is coordination of care and sharing of information. Medicine has become so complex that it is no longer possible for one doctor to provide all the services that are required by people with diseases that can affect multiple organs in various ways. Here is an opportunity to play an active role in your care and most doctors (and doctors' offices) will appreciate the contribution.

*Tip number 1*: Get copies of your own records and keep these in a file. It doesn't matter if you don't understand the terminology. You can read them if you like, but your role is really that of executive secretary. Do not rely on your doctor's office to send a copy. They say they will, and I am sure they mean it, but too many times the records are not sent, arrive too late, or are incomplete. Bring a copy with you, and do not give your only copy to the rheumatologist. Have the clerk make a copy on the spot and give you back your originals.

*Tip number 2*: Have the nurse put your records in your chart before the doctor sees you. It is time saving for the physician to have the laboratory tests from a previous workup on the same day that he or she does the history and physical. I can often finalize my diagnosis and offer a plan of treatment if I have this information available on the same day I first see a patient. (Some people want a second opinion "fresh," that is, they do not want to bias the doctor based on previous opinions. That is okay, but be candid with your doctor about this. Even if you wish to do this, include copies of test results.)

*Tip number 3*: Identify the "quarterback." This is the doctor who is going to coordinate your care. This may be your general practitioner, your general internist, your rheumatologist, or another subspecialist. You have to be clear in your own mind, and it has to be made clear to your doctor, who is playing that role. For my scleroderma patients who need tests from other specialists, and who will likely get treatment based on the results of those tests, I want to be the one calling the shots.

When I send a patient to a pulmonologist (lung specialist) or other specialist, I want that doctor to do the evaluation and get back to me with the results before starting treatment. Usually when I refer a patient to them, I indicate that this is the arrangement. This is important to ensure that a medication from one doctor will not conflict with another or that a test recently done by one specialist will not be repeated by another.

*Tip number 4*: Make sure all your subspecialists have all the other doctors' reports. The best way to do this is to request a copy of each specialist's report to be sent to you directly. It is okay to do this, and people do it all the time. You are not meddling or being nosy. There is nothing secret in the reports. If you are afraid that there will be something in the report that will frighten you, don't read it. If you do read it and get alarmed, talk to your doctor about it. You can also ask the specialist to send a copy of the report to all your doctors. This does not involve much extra work on the doctor's part (the same letter gets sent), and the only added expense is the mailing cost. It is very helpful for you to have a typed list of the names and addresses of all your doctors, or a business card from all the doctors who are to get reports. Pick up a couple of extra cards when you go to a new doctor. In any event, make sure you get a copy of the report for your personal file. You may be referred to some new specialist in the future, and having your own copies would be helpful.

Keep in mind that all your body systems are interrelated. The results of the lung workup will be relevant to the heart doctor and the GI doctor. Sometimes they may only glance at them for a second and put them down again. Sometimes all they need to see is the bottom of the report, where it says "normal." It does not take much time to read this, but the information is extremely valuable.

*Tip number 5*: It is not necessary in most situations to have the specialist call your primary doctor. This kind of communication is usually done by letter, which is dictated on the same day that you are seen. The problem is not with making a phone call; the problem is with playing phone tag for days in a row.

*Tip number 6*: You, your primary-care doctor, and your rheumatologist are going to have a long-term relationship. Figure out who in the office is the person who handles referrals and is the one who can get the doctor's attention. This may be the office manager, the receptionist, or the nurse. Before you run into problems, find out when the best time is to call and when the doctor is likely to call back. Some doctors make return calls at lunch or in the evening. If you are having a problem, call as early in the day as possible so that you can get on the list of people to call back.

### *Whom to Call*

Let us assume that you get sick with something. You have at least four, sometimes five doctors (primary-care physician, rheumatologist, pulmonologist, gastroenterologist, cardiologist) to choose from. This can be tricky, and the bottom line is that you have to make your own judgment call. If you really feel that the problem would be best addressed by, say, your rheumatologist but your insurance requires that you first contact your primary-care physician, call the primary-care person and ask immediately, over the phone, for a one-time extra referral. As you become more experienced with your condition, it will become easier and easier to make these decisions.

### The Emergency Room

If you experience trouble breathing, chest pain, or high fevers, go to the emergency room (ER). If these problems start during the day, notify your doctor's office first. If you have a choice, go to the emergency room of the hospital where your doctor is on staff. In most other situations, avoid the ER. They do not understand scleroderma. You will spend at least four hours there, and they are likely to send you home with instructions to call your doctor.

In summary, your doctor wants to provide you with the best care in the most timely and cost-efficient manner. Likewise, you want to receive the best care, and you don't want to undergo tests over and over again because the prior test results are unavailable and your doctor can't proceed with treatment without knowing these results. On the other hand, you want to be sure that the proper tests are done so that problems can be identified early and treated as well as possible. This is going to take some effort on your part. Following the tips above and being an active participant in your own care will go a long way toward making sure that this happens. You and your doctor are partners in this endeavor.

# 17

**❋ ❋ ❋**

# LIVING AN
# UNPREDICTABLE LIFE
# FACING AN
# UNCERTAIN FUTURE

What is different about you the day after your disease was diagnosed from you the day before? For many people, what has changed is their sense of mortality, of vulnerability, of order in life—basically their sense of the future.

A diagnosis of a rare, chronic, incurable illness brings you up short. You are not in control, and it is this lack of control that is at the heart of the difficulty for many people. I try to point out to patients that in reality they have never been in control of much that happens inside their bodies, and indeed in their lives. In actuality, though, most of us live every day as if we are in control, and we plan for a future that is predictable on a day-to-day basis. It is not possible to live an organized and effective life without this attitude. We go to the grocery store and plan dinners for the coming week. We worry about paying the bills and taking care of aging parents. In terms of the long run, we make the assumption that we or our spouse will work until retirement, that we will get the kids through school, and that we will be taking a vacation next summer. Although we may have known people with serious illnesses that disrupted their life plans, they are not us. We usually feel that such illnesses aren't supposed to happen to us.

Suddenly all that predictability has changed. How can you continue to live an organized and effective life in the face of this uncertainty?

## Living an Unpredictable Life

On hearing the diagnosis of scleroderma for the first time, people respond in many different ways. Some people want to get as much information as possible right from the beginning, while others are content to go from visit to visit without giving much thought to the future. Most people want to know what they can expect from the disease. They want to know what is going to happen to them in the future. Most people also need time initially to summon the emotional strength to ask the "big" questions: "Will I die from this? Will I be disabled?" Sometimes these questions remain unasked, since people are afraid of the answers.

Although these are all simple and straightforward questions, the answers are not. Scleroderma has such a variable course from one person to the next that it is very difficult to predict what will happen to any individual patient. The course varies from mild disease in some cases to very severe disease in others. Sometimes people who start out with very active and progressive disease reach a plateau and then slowly improve and do well in the long run.

There are some generalizations that can be made, however, about the pace and course of disease activity. The skin thickening tends to reach its maximum point in the first two to five years. Then it usually reaches a stable stage and sometimes will improve even without treatment. The onset of internal organ involvement, on the other hand, is highly unpredictable. Lung and gastrointestinal involvement tends to happen within the first few years but can occur at any time. Over and over again, patients tell me that they developed a complication (such as kidney disease) ten years or more after the diagnosis and that their doctors had told them it was not supposed to happen after the first five years. For the most part, I no longer try to predict a patient's outcome. I treat the disease as it currently exists. I monitor tests for the development or worsening of internal organ involvement, and I treat problems as they arise.

Because of the differences among individual patients and even at different times in the same patient, I cannot give a straight answer to questions such as "How long will I be able to keep on working?" Many of my patients continue to work, but this depends to some extent on the type of job they hold. There is a future after the diagnosis. It simply may not be the one you had planned. It may be worse, but it in some ways it may be better. Perhaps I can best illustrate this with some stories concerning real patients.

One of my patients had a job at the airport collecting money for parking. She worked in a small outdoor booth (in Michigan) and had to extend her hand out the window to every passing car. Although the booth was heated in the winter (in Michigan the cold weather begins in September and ends in May), the window was usually open and she could not avoid cold exposure. This in-and-out exposure was disastrous for a scleroderma patient with Raynaud's phenomenon and a tendency to get recurrent finger ulcers. In her case, she did have to change her job.

Another of my patients is a piano teacher. The first doctor she saw told her to stop playing the piano, since it would cause too much pressure on her fingertips. She was devastated and became depressed. When I saw her, I realized that she had limited, mild scleroderma, and as long as she did not have an open ulcer on her finger, I saw no reason for her not to resume playing. The exercise was actually good for her hands. That was more than ten years ago. She and her husband are now retired, and she has voluntarily stopped teaching but still plays for her own enjoyment and that of her family.

Another of my patients, a young man, was a construction worker and, of course, was outdoors most of the time. He was unable to continue work due to intolerance to cold and to the clumsiness of his hands from the numbness that cold exposure caused—he said he could barely hold a hammer in the cold, much less use it well.

My oldest patient is currently 93 years old. She was diagnosed at the age of 50. She sometimes uses a cane when she walks, to assist her balance, but gets around very well. She has outlived her husband and two of her doctors. Scleroderma has not interfered very much in her lifestyle over the past 43 years, except she has had to make a few more adjustments to the cold more than she otherwise might have done.

Another one of my patients, a middle-aged man with a desk job for one of the car companies in Detroit, told me the following story. At the height of his illness—and he had diffuse disease, with a lot of thick and tight skin on his hands, arms, face, trunk, and legs—his wife and daughter had to help him dress in the morning, especially to tie his shoes, since he could not bend over far enough to get his feet close to his hands, and he could not manipulate the laces to tie a tight bow. He said that one of his fears was that his shoes would become untied at work and he would be too embarrassed to ask a co-worker to tie them for him. He continued to go to work every day, both on days when he felt good and on days when he felt awful. That was eight years ago. Over time and with medication, his skin softened and he regained a lot of his flexibility. Even though he was getting better, he decided to take early retirement (at age 60) to spend more time with his family. He has not developed significant internal organ involvement. I don't see him in my office much anymore, since he is doing so well.

I have a patient who is a teacher in a middle school (sixth, seventh, and eighth grades). At the beginning of every school year she explains to her class why her hands look the way they do, why her fingers are so crooked. She lets them know that she will sometimes ask them for help with something she can't do. She tells me that she has no difficulty getting students to help out, but that still, after several years of explaining her situation to her students, it is tough every September.

One of my most heartbreaking cases was a young woman with a 12-year-old son and a devoted husband. Prior to her illness she had been primarily a homemaker but had taught some aerobics classes and did some hair styling for extra income. Five years after the scleroderma was diagnosed she was mostly bedridden. Her husband had to pick her up from bed to sit her up in the chair. She became unable to walk because her knees did not straighten out, and unable to comb her hair because she couldn't raise her arm at the shoulder high enough to reach. She died about three years ago. There is no way I can paint a rosy picture of this situation. I marveled at their fortitude and I admired their courage.

Every patient's story is different. Some of these stories are happy; some are tragic. Often the stories are a combination of the two. Most of my patients do not see themselves as courageous or extraordinary in any way. Rather, they see themselves as coping the best they can with the choices available to them.

How individuals respond emotionally and psychologically to their condition is a reflection of their underlying personality and all the life experiences they have had up to that point. People who have a tendency toward depression may become more depressed. People with a high degree of underlying anxiety will respond with greater nervousness and agitation. Some individuals, most commonly but not exclusively men, have difficulty dealing with feelings and may respond by becoming more distant and withdrawn. People with a strong sense of responsibility may see their illness as a failure to provide for their families.

All human beings resent sudden and undeserved loss. We all fear death and disability, and few of us are very enthusiastic about the unknown. There is no one "right" way to cope with your disease; you have to develop the way that suits you best.

The bookstores are filled with volumes on self-help and pop psychology. For the most part, these are uplifting and helpful. But there are some popular myths that may get in the way of your ability to come to terms with this new level of unpredictability in life and with the new identity that it brings. The following are several popular myths that I think are particularly harmful.

*Myth number 1*: You are in control of your body; whether you have mild disease or severe disease depends on how you respond to it.

*Response*: Whether you have mild disease or severe disease depends on your genetic predisposition to the disease and the level of the "triggering" factor (whatever the cause) you were exposed to. No amount of positive thinking will make scleroderma magically disappear. However, you may have more control than you realize over how you are affected by the disease. In this case, the key point is to appreciate the difference between pain and suffering.

Pain is the physiological response to a hurtful stimulus. This is necessary for survival to make sure that individuals avoid injury. Suffering, on the other hand, is the emotional and psychological response to pain or any unpleasant situation. Pain is always worse at night, when there are no distractions to keep our minds off the problem and when fatigue is added to the sensation of pain. The extent to which pain bothers us depends on what else is going on. A paper cut can be a mild annoyance if we are engaged in a really exciting activity, such as watching a favorite sports team win a very close match, or it can be a major discomfort if we are preparing our taxes and it is April 15. Perhaps the worst suffering is experienced not even by the person having the pain, but by a loved one who feels he or she can only stand by helplessly and watch.

Suffering is made worse by many things. Anxiety over not knowing where the pain is coming from can turn an episode of heartburn into an imaginary heart attack. Becoming more informed about your condition is a good way to deal with this type of anxiety. Although you may not like what the answer is, at least you will know the facts. I frequently see patients who are referred for the purpose of confirming the diagnosis of scleroderma. Even when I tell them that the suspicion of their doctor is correct and that they do, in fact, have scleroderma, they frequently express a sense of relief, since now they have a name for their condition, a reason that they are having all these strange symptoms, and an approach to treatment that makes sense. Fear of the unknown is almost always worse than knowing the true situation.

For some people, the most important source of suffering is the fear of loss—loss of function if the hands are involved, loss of importance if livelihood is interrupted, loss of identity as homemaker or breadwinner, loss of physical attractiveness. How do you get in control of this fear?

The key issue is one of identity. Identity changes throughout life, but most of the time these changes are gradual and fairly predictable. Having survived the great adolescent identity crisis, most people are still shocked at the change in their identity after the birth of their first child. Middle age happens very gradually and should come as a surprise to no one, but nonetheless gray hairs and wrinkles are seldom welcome. Retirement is a huge emotional transition for many people, even though it is quite predictable. Developing scleroderma also brings an identity crisis, made worse by its totally unexpected occurrence and by its complete unfamiliarity. A diagnosis makes many people feel as if they have changed from Jane Doe, teacher and mother of two, to Jane Doe, scleroderma patient. You are not your disease, but you are changed by it.

The first step in handling the situation, and thereby regaining emotional equilibrium, is to accept the idea that a change in identity, that is, a change in self-perception, is occurring. There is a "new you," and like the previous new yous of grown-up or parent or retiree, this transition is a process that occurs over an extended period of time. You also don't become a new you in a vacuum; your change in self-perception is influenced by your loved ones—spouse, children, friends. Unless they are brought along in this process, they will continue to expect the old you. You will probably need help in convincing them that the old you isn't around anymore. They may desperately want the old you to remain because they too are afraid of the unknown. There is frequently resentment over the fact that although you have the disease, they have to make changes. But people who really love you will change. Open communication, perhaps with the help of a family counselor, priest, minister, or rabbi, can make all the difference in the world.

*Myth number 2*: All life experiences are an opportunity for growth.

*Response*: Getting a diagnosis of a chronic, possibly debilitating disease is not good news, and no matter how your rephrase it, it is very difficult to see it as an opportunity. A true opportunity is one that, if you had to live your life over, you would freely choose again, although the benefits may not have been apparent at the time. An example of this tragedy-turned-opportunity is most often seen in individuals who have lost their job and who then go through a difficult time of reassessment, discover their true calling, and end up much more satisfied than if they had remained in their original, secure, but unfulfilling occupation. I have never had a scleroderma patient, even those who do quite well, describe their situation as a true opportunity. The fact is that some life experiences are bad, and personal growth can be very painful.

However, I have had many patients tell me how scleroderma forced them to reevaluate their lives and their priorities. Rather than being caught up on the treadmill of jobs and responsibilities, they stepped back and decided what was truly important. This is almost always family and relationships. They become aware that their most precious gift is time spent with loved ones.

Family members and loved ones have to be let in, not kept out. Isolation is damaging to the patient and devastating to any relationship. Family counseling may be necessary to assist in this process. Family members may feel lost and abandoned and just as out of control of the situation as the patient. Having a neutral person with whom to discuss these feelings and a safe environment in which to bring them up are important parts of keeping open the lines of communication.

As strange as it may sound, some relationships deepen and are strengthened by dealing with this adversity. I want to emphasize that I am not asking you to be happy about having scleroderma; rather, I am suggesting that you can use this to develop a better understanding of yourself and a deeper relationship with your loved ones.

### The Difference between "Suffering From" and "Living With"

There is a difference between being a victim suffering from a disease and being a person living with a condition. The difference is more than just attitude. The term "victim" is fraught with a sense of passivity and helplessness. It brings to mind individuals whose lives were overrun by forces so much more powerful than they that they had no hope of influencing their own fate. On the other hand, the term "person living with ..." implies an individual identity influenced but not overwhelmed by the condition. It combines a sense of acceptance of the condition (after all, there is no choice) with the notion that the person has an identity other than that defined by the disease. It should be clear that I prefer the second designation. The point is that although the disease may change your self-perception, it does not have to dominate your existence.

*Myth number 3*: We all face an uncertain future; your situation is no different from that of anyone else.

*Response*: The weather is uncertain, but the fact that the sun will come up tomorrow is considered a sure bet. Human beings get used to a particular level of certainty, which permits them to structure their lives accordingly. A diagnosis of an incurable disease, especially one with an uncertain prognosis or outcome, introduces a level of uncertainty that is above and beyond the usual level we live with, and does indeed represent a new reality. People get used to a greater level of uncertainty.

In my practice I have noticed that people with a new diagnosis of scleroderma have a great many questions in the beginning. I can answer the trivial ones ("Why am I stiff? Why do I have heartburn?"), but I cannot answer the important ones ("What causes scleroderma? What is the cure?"). After a while, people have fewer questions as they become more familiar with and more knowledgeable about their own condition.

## Where to Get Help

The Scleroderma Foundation has chapters and support groups around the country. Appendix 2 lists the foundation's contact information as well as other organizations that provide support and information.

✳ ✳ ✳

This book ends with a view to the future. We now know more about scleroderma than ever before. Research continues daily, and progress, though slow, is clearly being made. New treatments are being developed to better deal with symptoms, prevent progression, and improve well-being. One day the cause will be known and the cure will be found.

# Appendix 1
✳ ✳ ✳

# CRITERIA FOR THE CLASSIFICATION OF SYSTEMIC SCLERODERMA

## *American College of Rheumatology*

### *Major Criterion:*

Skin thickness of the fingers plus skin thickness extending over the back of the hand.

### *Minor Criteria:*

1. Skin thickness of the fingers (sclerodactyly)
2. Pulmonary fibrosis in the bases of the lungs
3. Digital pitting scars, ulcers, or loss of finger pad substance

A diagnosis of scleroderma is considered definite if either the single major criterion is present, or if at least two of the three minor criteria are present.

Localized forms of scleroderma and sclerodermalike disorders are excluded from these criteria.

Adapted from A. T. Masi, G. P. Rodnan, T. A. Medsger Jr., et al., Preliminary criteria for the classification of systemic sclerosis (scleroderma). *Arthritis and Rheumatism 23* (1980): 581–90.

# Appendix 2
✳ ✳ ✳

# SCLERODERMA SUPPORT GROUPS AND RESOURCE MATERIAL

*U.S. Patient Support and Information*

**Arthritis Foundation**
National office: 1314 Spring St., NW
Atlanta, GA 30309
Telephone: 404-872-7100 or 800-283-7800
   The Arthritis Foundation has local chapters throughout the United States and has literature on all the connective tissue diseases, including scleroderma. The Arthritis Foundation raises funds for research on all these diseases.

   Scleroderma Clinical Trials Consortium web site: sctc-online.org. This website contains a list of current scleroderma clinical trials with contact information

**Scleroderma Foundation**
INSERT NEW ADDRESS
Telephone: 800-722-4673 or 978-750-4499
Fax: 978-750-9902
E-mail: sclerofed@aol.com
World Wide Web address: http://www.scleroderma.com
   The Scleroderma Foundation has local chapters and support groups throughout the United States and has affiliated groups in Canada. The foundation raises funds for research, publishes literature on scleroderma, sponsors conferences, and conducts public awareness campaigns.

**Scleroderma Research Foundation**
INSERT NEW ADDRESS
2320 Bath Street, Suite 315
Santa Barbara, CA 93105
Telephone: 805-563-9133 or 800-441-CURE
World Wide Web address: http://www.srfcure.org
   This foundation also raises funds to support research.

**National Institutes of Health (NIH) /
National Institute of Arthritis, Musculoskeletal,
and Skin Diseases (NIAMS)**
1 AMS Circle
Bethesda, MD 20892-3675
Telephone: 301-495-4484
Fax: 301-718-6366
World Wide Web address: http://www.nih.gov/niams/
   National Arthritis and Musculoskeletal and Skin Diseases Information Clearinghouse, a public service sponsored by the National Institute of Arthritis and Musculoskeletal and Skin Diseases (NIAMS) of the National Institutes of Health (NIH). The Clearinghouse distributes National Institute of Arthritis and Musculoskeletal and Skin Diseases publications; it also maintains a file in the Combined Health Information Database (CHID), publicly accessible on the Internet. Materials indexed in CHID include books, pamphlets, journal articles, and audiovisuals. Personal information requests are fulfilled by Information Specialists and referred to other appropriate organizations for additional information.

## Outside the United States

**Raynaud's and Scleroderma Association**
LOOK UP NEW ADDRESS
112 Crewe Road
Alsager, Cheshire ST7 2JA
England
Telephone: 01270 872776
Fax: 01270 883556
E-mail: webmaster@raynauds.demon.co.uk
World Wide Web address: http://www.raynauds.demon.co.uk

**Associazione Patologie Autoimmuni**
Via degli Uliveti, 8
Silvi Marina
64029 Teremo Italy
Phone: 011 39 085.935.35.60

## Books and Pamphlets on Scleroderma Written for Patients

The following three books are all available from the Scleroderma Foundation (address listed above).

Mark Flapan, Perspectives on Living with Scleroderma. Scleroderma Federation, 1997.

E. Carwile LeRoy, M.D., Understanding and Managing Scleroderma. Scleroderma Federation, 1996.

Dana Lovvorn, Scleroderma: Surviving the Seventeen Year Itch. United Scleroderma Foundation, 1996.

## Literature and Resources on Scleroderma for Doctors

Philip J. Clements and Daniel E. Furst, eds., Systemic Sclerosis. X, Williams and Wilkins, 2004.

V. D. Steen, ed., "Scleroderma—Preface," introduction to a special issue on scleroderma, Rheumatic Disease Clinics of North America, vol. 22, no. 4, 1996. UPDATE THIS

Carol M. Black and Allen R. Myers, eds., Systemic Sclerosis (Scleroderma). Gower Medical Publishing, 1985.

Scleroderma Clinical Trials Consortium web site: sctc-online.org. This website contains a list of current scleroderma clinical trials with contact information

General Rheumatology Textbooks

William N. Kelly, et al., Textbook of Rheumatology, 4th ed. W. B. Saunders, 1996.

John H. Klippel and Paul A. Dieppe, Rheumatology, 2nd ed. Mosby, 1997.

Daniel J. McCarty and William J. Koopman, Arthritis and Allied Conditions: A Textbook of Rheumatology. Lea and Febiger, 1993.

# Glossary

✳ ✳ ✳

*Aldolase*: a muscle enzyme normally present in low levels in the blood, but elevated to high levels in conditions like polymyositis in which there is muscle inflammation

*Alveolitis*: inflammation of the small air sacs in the lungs

*Alveolus*, pl. *alveoli*: small air sac in the lung

*American College of Rheumatology (ACR)*: the professional organization of rheumatologists

*Anemia*: low number of red cells and/or low amount of hemoglobin in the blood

*Antibody*: a protein made by cells of the immune system that attacks a substance, usually a foreign substance, in the body

*Anticentromere antibody*: an antibody directed against a protein in the cell nucleus; it is found most often in patients with limited scleroderma but can be seen occasionally in other conditions

*Anti-DNA antibody*: an antibody directed against genetic material in the cell; it is usually seen in lupus patients and only rarely seen in scleroderma patients

*Antinuclear antibody (ANA)*: an antibody directed against one of the many components in the nucleus (internal compartment containing the genes) of the cell seen in most scleroderma and lupus patients, and occasionally seen in other disorders

*Antitopoisomerase antibody*: an antibody directed against an enzyme in the nucleus; it is also called the Scl-70 antibody and is seen in about 25 percent of scleroderma patients, usually those with diffuse skin involvement

*Arrhythmia*: abnormal heart rhythm

*Arthralgia*: pain in the joints

*Arthritis*: inflammation in the joints

*Atrial fibrillation*: a form of abnormal heart rhythm in which the heart beats in an irregular pattern

*Autoantibody*: a protein made by cells of the immune system that attacks the body's own tissues

*Autoimmune disease*: a disease in which the immune system attacks the body's own tissue, also called connective tissue disease; the most common autoimmune diseases are rheumatoid arthritis, lupus, scleroderma, polymyositis, and Sjogren's syndrome

*Autonomic nervous system*: that part of the nervous system that controls the inner workings of the body; it is divided into the sympathetic and parasympathetic systems

*Barrette's esophagus*: a precancerous change in the lining cells of the esophagus at the area near the stomach

*Bell's palsy*: weakness or paralysis of the muscles on one side of the face; also called seventh nerve palsy; a form of cranial neuropathy

*Biopsy*: the process of taking a small piece of tissue to examine under the microscope

*Bradycardia*: abnormally slow heart rhythm; also called *bradyarrhythmia*

*Broncho-alveolar lavage*: a procedure in which liquid is first introduced into one area of the lungs (through a bronchoscope) and then suctioned out to get samples of mucus and cells to determine whether there is infection, inflammation, or cancer

*Bronchoscopy*: a procedure in which a tube is passed into the lungs to visualize the airways and to obtain samples for analysis

*Bronchus*, pl. *bronchi*: large air tube in the lung

*BUN*: blood urea nitrogen, a substance in the blood that is one of the breakdown products of the body; it is normally excreted by the kidneys, so an abnormally high BUN suggests that the kidneys are not functioning well

*Calcinosis*: calcium deposits in the skin or just below the skin, commonly seen in scleroderma, but also occurring in some other diseases

*Calcium channel blocker*: a type of medication that results in opening up (dilatation) of the blood vessels, used to improve circulation, to lower blood pressure, or to treat some types of heart disease

*Capillary*: the smallest blood vessel in the body

*Cardiology*: the branch of medicine that treats heart disease

*Carpal tunnel syndrome*: numbness and tingling of the hand usually affecting the thumb, index and long fingers due to pressure on the median nerve at the wrist; this is one form of compression neuropathy

*Collagen*: a fibrous protein made by cells that provides the firmness in the skin, forms the lining of organs, and is the basic structural protein in bones, tendons, ligaments, and joints

*Colonoscopy*: a procedure of passing a tube into the colon to visualize the lining of the bowel and take samples of abnormal tissue

*Connective tissue diseases*: autoimmune diseases including rheumatoid arthritis, lupus, scleroderma, polymyositis, and Sjogren's syndrome

*Constriction*: narrowing

*Contracture*: persistent bent position of a joint, the inability to fully straighten out a joint

*Cortisone*: a powerful anti-inflammatory medication that occurs naturally, at low levels, in the body; a type of steroid

*CPK*: creatine phosphokinase, a muscle enzyme, the blood level of which is elevated when muscle is inflamed or damaged, for example, with heart muscle damage in a heart attack or with skeletal muscle damage in myositis

*Cranial neuropathy*: disease of one of the cranial nerves that provide sensation and muscle movement to the face and head

*Creatinine*: a substance in the blood that is abnormally high when the kidneys do not work well

*CREST*: an acronym that stands for calcinosis, Raynaud's phenomenon, esophageal dysfunction, sclerodactyly, and telangiectasia; describes a form of scleroderma

*Dermatology*: the branch of medicine that treats skin diseases

*Dermatomyositis*: a disease with inflammation of the muscles resulting in weakness, and inflammation of the skin, causing a rash

*Dermis*: the skin

*Dialysis*: use of a machine that cleanses the blood of waste products when the kidneys are unable to do so

*Digital pits*: tiny, indented areas in the fingertips that are typical of scleroderma

*Digital ulcers*: open sores on the fingers or toes

*Digits*: fingers and toes

*Dilate*: to open up

*DLCO*: diffusion in liters of carbon monoxide; a test that measures the ability of the lungs to get oxygen into the blood

*Duodenum*: the first part of the bowel after the stomach

*Dysphagia*: difficulty swallowing

*Dyspnea*: shortness of breath

*Echocardiogram*: an ultrasound test of the heart

*Edema*: swelling

*Edematous*: swollen

*Endocrinology*: the branch of medicine that treats diseases of the glands, such as thyroid disease and diabetes

*Endoscopy*: a procedure that involves passing a tube into the esophagus and stomach (upper endoscopy) or into the colon (lower endoscopy or colonoscopy) to visualize the bowel and sample abnormal tissue

*Entrapment neuropathy*: damage to a nerve due to pressure along its course; also known as compression neuropathy

*Eosinophilia myalgia syndrome (EMS)*: a condition characterized by muscle pain and inflammation, nerve inflammation, and increased eosinophils in the blood

*Eosinophilic fasciitis*: a sclerodermalike illness characterized by inflammation in the area just beneath the skin and fat, called the fascia

*Eosinophils*: one of the types of white blood cells; they are increased in some cases of scleroderma and in some of the sclerodermalike disorders

*Epidermis*: the outermost layer of the skin, specially adapted to provide protection against most injuries; injury limited to the epidermis does not result in a scar; examples of this are sunburns and shallow scratches; scleroderma is primarily a disease of the dermis, the lower layer of skin beneath the epidermis

*Esophagitis*: inflammation of the lining of the esophagus

*Esophagus*: the swallowing tube between the mouth and the stomach

*Fasciitis*: inflammation of the fascia, a layer that separates muscles from the overlying fat and skin

*Fibroblast*: a cell that makes collagen

*Fibrosis*: scar tissue buildup that replaces normal tissue

*Gastric Antral Vascular Ectasia (GAVE)*: dilated blood vessels in the stomach lining that can bleed

*Gastritis*: inflammation of the lining of the stomach

*Gastroenterology*: the branch of medicine that deals with digestive and liver problems

*Gastroesophageal reflux disease (GERD)*: a condition in which stomach acid passes up into the esophagus, usually causing heartburn and damage to the lining of the esophagus

*Gastroesophageal stricture*: a narrowing of the junction between the esophagus and the stomach, usually as a result of recurrent acid reflux, which causes scar tissue buildup

*Gastrointestinal tract (GI tract)*: the digestive system, including the esophagus, stomach, duodenum, small bowel, large bowel or colon, and rectum; it also includes the liver and gall bladder

*Graves' disease*: a thyroid condition usually characterized by an overactive thyroid gland

*H-2 blocker*: a type of medicine that decreases acid secretion in the stomach

*Hashimoto's disease* or *Hashimoto's thyroiditis*: a thyroid disease that usually results in an underactive thyroid

*Heart block*: a defect in the electrical system of the heart that can cause an abnormal pulse

*HLA test*: histocompatibility locus antigen test, a blood test to determine the genes that control the immune system; usually only done for research

*Holter monitor*: a portable instrument that measures heartbeat for an extended period of time (usually 24 hours) to detect abnormalities in the heart rate that occur intermittently

*Hyperpigmentation*: too much pigment, or darker-than-normal skin

*Hypopigmentation*: loss of pigment, or lighter-than-normal skin

*Infarction*: death of tissue from lack of blood supply

*Ischemia*: lowered blood supply

*Leucopenia*: abnormally low white blood cell count

*Linear scleroderma*: a form of localized scleroderma in which the thickened skin is in the pattern of a line on the face or down an arm or leg

*Lupus* or *systemic lupus erythematosus (SLE)*: an autoimmune disease characterized by inflammation in multiple organ systems, frequently involving skin, joints, and the kidneys

*Lymphocyte*: a type of white blood cell that is important in immunity

*Lymphopenia*: abnormally low lymphocyte count

*Malabsorption*: decreased absorption of nutrients in the bowel; in scleroderma this is due to decreased bowel motility and overgrowth of bacteria, resulting in diarrhea and weight loss

*Malignant phase hypertension*: a sudden and dangerous increase in blood pressure that can result in kidney failure if not treated

*MCTD*: mixed connective tissue disease, a disease characterized by features of lupus, scleroderma, and polymyositis, usually with a positive anti-RNP antibody test

*Morphea*: a form of localized scleroderma characterized by patches of thickened skin

*Myocardial infarction (MI)*: heart attack

*Myocarditis*: inflammation of the heart muscle

*Myopathy*: muscle abnormality

*Myositis*: muscle inflammation

*Neuralgia*: pain of the nerve

*Neuropathy*: damage to nerves

*Neuritis*: inflammation of nerves

*NIH*: National Institutes of Health—the federal agency, funded by Congress, that provides grants for most of the medical research in the U.S.; it consists of 11 separate institutes divided among diseases including arthritis, cancer, and kidney, lung, heart, nerve diseases, etc.

*NIAMS*: National Institute of Arthritis, Musculoskeletal and Skin Diseases; the section of the NIH that supports most of the scleroderma research as well as general rheumatology research in the U.S.

*Nonsteroidal anti-inflammatory drugs (NSAIDs)*: a class of medication that inhibits inflammation by decreasing prostaglandins

*Osteoarthritis*: a wear-and-tear arthritis, or degenerative arthritis, that occurs with age

*Osteoporosis*: thinning of bones due to loss of calcium

*Pacemaker*: a device that controls heart rhythm

*Parasympathetic nervous system*: part of the autonomic nervous system that controls the functioning of the internal organs

*Pericarditis*: inflammation of the sac that surrounds the heart

*Pericardium*: the sac that surrounds the heart

*Peristalsis*: the normal motility, or muscle activity, in the esophagus, stomach, and bowel

*Pigmentation*: skin color

*Pleurisy*: inflammation of the lining of the lungs, usually painful

*Polymyositis*: inflammation of the muscles

*Prednisone*: a form of cortisone or steroid hormone that is a powerful anti-inflammatory medication

*Primary biliary cirrhosis (PBC)*: scarring in the liver caused by damage to the small bile ducts, seen occasionally in scleroderma and not related to alcohol

*Prokinetic agent*: a medication that improves motility in the gut

*Proteinuria*: protein in the urine

*Proton pump inhibitor*: a medication that decreases stomach acid

*Pruritus*: itching

*Pulmonary fibrosis*: scar tissue buildup in the lungs that interferes with normal function

*Pulmonary function tests*: tests performed by blowing into an instrument that measures lung volume, airflow, and ability to get oxygen into the blood

*Pulmonary hypertension*: high blood pressure in the pulmonary arteries; this can occur in the absence of high blood pressure as measured in the arm

*Pulmonology*: the branch of medicine that treats lung diseases

*Raynaud's phenomenon*: color changes of the fingers on cold exposure, usually white, then blue, then red; if it occurs alone it is called primary Raynaud's disease; if it occurs with scleroderma or lupus, it is called secondary Raynaud's phenomenon

*Reflux*: usually referring to gastroesophageal reflux, the backflow of acid from the stomach into the esophagus

*Rheumatoid arthritis*: an inflammatory autoimmune arthritis of multiple joints characterized by joint deformity and destruction

*Rheumatology*: the branch of medicine that treats all forms of arthritis and the autoimmune diseases

*Sclerodactyly*: thickening of the skin of the fingers

*Sclerosis*: hardening

*Scl-70*: an autoantibody in the blood that occurs in about 25 percent of scleroderma patients and usually is found in those with diffuse skin disease; also known as antitopoisomerase antibody

*SLE*: systemic lupus erythematosus (see lupus)

*Steroid*: a class of hormone that is either anti-inflammatory (glucocorticoids, cortisone, prednisone) or one of the sex hormones (estrogen or testosterone)

*Stricture*: narrowing

*Subcutaneous*: under the skin

*Sympathetic nervous system*: part of the autonomic nervous system that controls the function of internal organs

*Telangiectasias*: small red spots on the skin due to enlargement of tiny blood vessels

*Tendonitis*: inflammation of tendons

*Tendon rub*: a sound like rubbing two pieces of leather together, made by the motion of a tendon in an inflamed tendon sheath; it is characteristic of scleroderma but can also occur after injury to a tendon

*Thrombocytopenia*: abnormally low platelets

*Thrombocytosis*: abnormally high platelets

*Total parenteral nutrition (TPN)*: a form of feeding through veins for individuals who cannot maintain nutrition by eating

*Watermelon stomach*: a striped appearance of the lining of the stomach due to thinning of the mucous layer and dilatation of the underlying blood vessels; it frequently is associated with bleeding from these blood vessels; also called gastric antral vascular ectasia (GAVE)

# Index

✳ ✳ ✳